영어권 의료관광 서류의 번역과 작성

본 과제(결과물)는 교육과학기술부의 재원으로 한국연구재단의 지원을 받아 수행된 광역경제권 선도산업 인재양성사업의 연구결과입니다.

영어권 의료관광 서류의 번역과 작성

| 주영탁 지음 |

小花

머리말

우리나라가 의료관광 사업을 국가적 차원에서 적극적으로 지원하고 의료서비스상품 개발과 마케팅 등 여러 가지 사업을 추진하면서 국내 의료 시설을 찾는 외국인의 수가 꾸준히 늘어나고 있습니다. 아직까지 여러 가지 과제들이 많이 남아 있지만 우리나라의 우수한 의료진과 의학 기술이 세계적으로 알려지고 인정받게 되는 현상에 비추어 볼 때 앞으로 더욱 많은 외국인들을 유치할 수 있을 것이라고 생각합니다.

필자는 한림대학교에서 펼친 의료관광 인재양성 사업의 일환으로 영어권 통·번역 수업을 맡으면서, 실제 외국인 진료 상황을 파악하고자 몇몇 국내 대형 병원의 국제 진료부를 직접 방문하여 현장의 의료진으로부터 고충과 시급하게 해결해야 할 문제들이 아직 많이 산재해 있음을 절감할 수 있었습니다.

모든 의료관광 사업과 관련하여 필요한 여러 가지 서류들을 작성하고, 각 나라의 해당 언어별로 번역하여 문서화하는 것은 이 서비스 산업에서 가장 기본이 되는 작업입니다. 의료서비스에 관련된 문서들은 그 자체가 법적 효력을 갖게 되며, 외국인 환자 유치에 있어 서비스의 질을 높이고, 여러 가지 사고나 법적 분쟁을 막을 수 있는 매우 중요하고 필수적인 요소이기 때문입니다.

이 책에서는 진료에 관계되는 서류를 중점적으로 다루었고, 기본적인 내용을 다양하게 다루고자 여러 가지 실제 서류들을 소개하였습니다. 병원을 찾는 외국인은 무엇보다 의사소통이 원활해야 할 뿐 아니라, 모든 정보를 문서화하여 보관할 수 있도록 해 주어야 합니다. 국내에서 이루어진 모든 진료 내용을 담은 환자 차트도 해당 언어로 번역해서 제공해 주어야 합니다.

이러한 작업을 하는 데 적용할 수 있는 여러 가지 서류와 그 형식, 번역에 사용되는 용어들과 올바른 사용법 등을 정리해 보았습니다.

이 책을 쓰기 시작하면서 1989년 처음 병원에서 일을 맡게 되었을 때 생각이 났습니다. 한 달간의 인턴 일정에서, 병원 관계 일 전반을 배울 수 있었는데, 그때는 지금처럼 문서들이 전자 문서화되기 전이었고, 일일이 손으로 기록하여 파일 형식으로 보관하였습니다. 이제 시대는 변했지만, 기록 및 문서화 보관의 중요성은 변치 않습니다.

앞으로 펼쳐질 의료관광 사업에 동참할 많은 통·번역사들에게 조금이나마 도움이 되기를 바랍니다.

2012년 1월

주영탁

차례

I. 의료관광 서류

의료관광 서류란 의료관광 서비스 과정에 필요한 모든 문서를 포함한다. 그 종류를 살펴보면 다음과 같다.

1. 상담 관련 서류

상담 신청서: 치료받고자 하는 내용, 인적사항, 현재 상태, 과거 병력 및 치료내역, 약의 복용 이력, 특이한 사항들

예상되는 치료, 관광 계획 및 견적서

환자에게 필요한 자료 요청서: 진단서, 검사 기록 등

2. 계약서

환자 보험관계 서류

지불 능력에 대한 증명서

지불에 대한 여러 가지 서류들

예약 확인서

3. 입국절차 관련 서류

입국목적 사실 확인서

유치의료기관 등록증

비자 관련 업무 매뉴얼

입국 준비사항 설명 및 안내서

호텔 예약에 관계되는 서류

4. 의료 서류

1) 환자 접수에 필요한 서류 (Patient Information & Sign-in Sheet)
2) 환자 문진표(Patient Questionnaire): 환자의 모든 신상, 과거 병력, 건강상태(Comprehensive Review of Patients Medical History and Physical Exam), 보험정보(Insurance Information) 등에 대한 내용이 들어 있다.
3) 환자 진료 및 경과기록지(Patient Medical Chart Notes and Progress Note)
4) 각종동의서(Consents): 진찰 및 치료동의서, 환자 의료기록 사용동의서, 검사동의서, 수술동의서 등이 포함된다.
5) 각종 진료 관계 서류들(Miscellaneous Medical Reports)
   - □ 수술 기록지(Operative Report)
   - □ 병리과 보고서(Pathology Report)
   - □ 방사선 치료에 대한 상담 기록지(Radiation Therapy Consultation Note)
6) 각종 검사 안내문(Brochure)
7) 의뢰서(Referral) 및 소견서(Letters: Email, Memos…)
8) 설명서(Information, Instruction)

5. 퇴원 서류

1) 퇴원보고서(Discharge Summary)
2) 해당국가 보험 청구서 발급
3) 귀국 후 주의 사항 안내서 등

6. 출국 서류

출국절차 안내서

7. 사후 관리

연락하는 데 필요한 정보 안내서
온라인 커뮤니케이션에 필요한 서류양식들

이 외에도 여러 가지 상황에 따라 다양하고 더 많은 서류들이 필요하게 된다. 따라서 의료관광에 관계되는 광범위한 서류들을 전부 다룰 수는 없고, 이 책에서는 4번에 해당하는 병원접수에서부터 진찰, 입원, 검사, 여러 가지 시술 등에 필요한 병원에서 쓰이는 서류들만을 다루었다.

II. 의료기록(Medical Record)

환자의 의료기록은 일정 체계에 따라 작성되며, 진료와 관계되는 모든 내용을 포함한다. 이 내용은 철저히 환자의 개인정보이며, 따라서 도덕적, 법적으로 그 내용이 보호를 받아야만 한다. 따라서 환자의 정보가 어떤 경우에 노출되어 사용될 수 있는지, 어떻게 보관되고 어떻게 파기될 수 있는지에 대한 일정한 계약 또는 법의 적용이 필요하다. 의료기록은 문서로 기록되기도 하고, 전자 의료기록(electronic record system)도 있다.

1. 환자의 의료기록(Medical Record)

환자의 의료기록은 일정 체계에 따라 작성되며, 환자의 모든 의료에 관계되는 내용을 포함하는 기록부이다. 이것은 철저히 환자의 개인 정보이며, 따라서 도덕적으로, 법적으로 그 내용이 보호를 받아야만 한다. 즉, 환자의 정보가 어떤 경우에 노출되어 사용될 수 있는지, 어떻게 보관되고 어떻게 파기될 수 있는지에 대한 일정한 계약 또는 법의 적용이 필요하다.

의료기록은 문서로 기록되기도 하고, 전자 의료기록(electronic record system)도 있다. 전자 의료기록은 현재 보편화되어 어느 의료기관에서든 전자 문서 형태로 환자정보를 기록·보관한다. 환자 자신의 정보 접근이 용이할 뿐 아니라, 환자가 다수의 의료진에게 진찰 및 진료를 받을 경우 여러 곳에서 다발적으로 정보를 쉽고 빠르게 공유할 수 있다. 또한 필요에 따라서 문서는 스캔(scan)하여 보관할 수도 있다. 모든 환자 정보는 일어나자마자, 바로 그 장소에서 기록하는 것이 원칙이다. 그리고 그때그때마다 번역되어 외국인 환자와 그 가족에게 제공되어야겠다. 최근에는 USB에 모든 정보를 보관해 환자가 항상 소지할 수 있도록 간편하게 만들어져(portable electronic medical record) 응급 시 손쉽게 정보에 접근할 수 있도록 하였다. 문서로 된 기록은 대개 의료기관에서 보관하고 있지만, 최근에 와서 환자 개인이 직접 보관하는 사례가 많아지고 있다.

2. 의료기록의 내용

1) 환자정보

각 의료기관의 의료서비스 종류에 따라 내용이 달라질 수 있지만, 보통 환자의 신상에 대한 내용, 과거, 현재의 병력, 검사 및 그 결과, 복용약, 추천서, 환자에게 제공된 모든 자료 등을 모두 포함한다. 때로 환자의 지불 관계에 대한 내용도 포함된다.

환자의 개인 신상정보로 주소, 전화번호, 환자 고유 번호 등 환자에 대한 정보 및 인종, 종교에 대한 것 등까지 포함할 수 있다. 응급 시 접촉할 수 있는 사람의 성명 및 전화번호도 포함한다.

□ 환자의 모든 병력
□ 외과적 치료 경력
□ 수술내용, 수술 경위, 담당의의 시술내용
□ 산과적 경력: 임신 및 출산
□ 약물 복용 및 약물에 대한 알레르기
□ 현재 및 과거에 복용한 약품에 대한 정보, 약물에 대한 알레르기 반응
□ 가족력(Family history)
□ 가족의 병력, 사망 원인, 유전병 유무
□ 속해 있는 사회와의 관계
□ 환자의 인간관계, 사회에 대한 기대, 경력, 학력, 종교 등: 환자의 생활 전반 조건이 건강에 어떤 영향을 끼치는가를 알 수 있는 실마리가 될 수 있다.
□ 습관: 흡연, 음주습관, 운동, 식습관, 혹은 성생활 등 건강에 영향을 끼칠 수 있는 요소들
□ 예방접종에 대한 기록: 예방 접종 및 면역에 대한 기록
□ 성장 기록(Growth chart): 어린이 및 청년의 성장에 대한 기록, 병력, 사회적 스트레스 행동발달 상황도 포함된다.

2) 의료기록(Medical Chart Note)

□ 치료받고자 하는 증세(Chief complaint)

□ 증세의 내용 및 기간 등(Symptom and sign)

□ 현재 앓고 있는 병(History of the present illness)

□ 진찰(Physical examination)기록

생체 사인(체온, 맥박, 혈압, 호흡수), 근육계, 내장기관 등 환자의 증세와 관계있는 신체 기관에 대한 조사(사지의 움직임) 평가 및 계획(Assessment and plan), 병에 대한 평가 요약, 진단명과 그에 따른 치료 내용

□ 의사의 지시(Orders)

의사의 지시사항, 의료진이 의료진에게 보내는 지시사항, 치료 진행상황 기록(Progress notes), 환자의 치료상황을 날짜별로 정리한다(Daily updates).

□ 검사결과(Test results)

모든 검사 그리고 병리학적 검사의 결과, 그 외 모든 병력, 임플란트 경력, 약물치료, 중환자실 입원 경력 등과 복용(약, 음료, 영양분, 물, 수혈) 및 배설물(출혈, 배뇨, 배설물, 구토, 땀), 동공 크기 관찰 등을 기록한다.

3. 관리상의 문제

1) 기록의 소유권, 기록의 개방 및 접근성, 폐기 등 법적 문제

□ 작성(Production)

- 작성 시 주의사항: 지울 수 없는 펜을 사용해야 하며, 오류가 있을 때는 반드시 지우지 말고, 줄을 그어서 변경하고 그 부분에 사인을 해야 한다.
- 작성은 다음과 같은 의료진 및 그 관계자만 작성에 참여할 수 있다: 의사, 간호사, 응급실 의료진, 인턴, 통역사, 물리치료사, 약사, 의료조무사, 언어치료사, 레지던트, 영양사 등

□ 소유권(Ownership)

기본적으로 환자의 소유이지만 의료기관에서 보관하게 된다. 환자는 자신의 의료기록이 정확하게 기록되어 있는지 확인하고, 오류에 대해서 의료진에게 정정을 요구할 수 있다. 영국에서는 National Health Service 산하 모든 환자 기록은 모두 보건국에 판권에 대한 권리가 있다.

□ 접근성(Accessibility)

미국에서는 환자 자신과 환자를 돌보는 의료진에게만 국한된 것을 원칙으로 한다. 단, 환자가 동의한 경우에 한해서 제3자에게 권리를 줄 수도 있다. 미국에서는 1996년 건강보험 이동성 및 책임법인 HIPAA(Health Insurance Portability and Accountability Act)를 제정했으며 이 법률의 목적은 개인의 동의 없이는 누구에게도 공개되지 않도록 개인 건강 정보를 보호하는 법이다.

전자 정보로 보관된 환자의 정보는 아이디, 비밀번호 등을 통해 환자 자신(또는 법적인 권리를 갖는 자)과 법적으로 한정되어 있는 의료진만 접근할 수 있도록 한다.

□ 자격(Capacities)

환자가 미성년자인 경우에 합법적 보호자가 환자를 대신하여 권리를 수행할 수 있다. 그 외 정신 질환자, 중독 환자, 혼수상태의 환자 등에 관해 법적보호자에게 권리가 주어진다.

□ 응급 상황 시(Medical emergency)

환자와 직접적인 대화가 어려울 경우 환자 의무 기록은 특정 동의 절차 없이 의료진에 의해 사용될 수 있다. 단, 미리 환자가 그런 상황을 위해 준비한 법적 서류가 있다면 문제될 것이 없다.

□ 연구, 감사 및 평가(Research, auditing, and evaluation)

의료 관련 연구, 재정 감사, 프로그램 평가 등을 위해 쓰일 수도 있다.

그러나 환자의 직접적 신상에 대한 노출은 금지되어 있다.

□ 사망 또는 손상의 위험이 있을 때(Risk of death or harm)

환자의 사망이나 손상을 가져오게 될 위험이 있는 상황에서 환자의 동의 없이 쓰일 수 있다. 단, 환자에 대한 기록내용을 다른 목적에 이용할 수 없다(예: 환자가 마약 등을 소유한 혐의가 드러나게 되더라도 환자에 대한 기록을 법적으로 응징하는 데 쓸 수는 없다).

2) 문서의 파기(Destruction)

환자 의료기록서는 특정 기간 동안 보존되어야 한다. 영국의 경우, 어떤 문제가 제기될 경우 환자가 살아 있는 동안의 모든 기록이 요구되며, 모든 기록 정보를 7년간 보존하는 것을 원칙으로 하고 있다. 또한 어린이의 경우 20세에 도달할 때까지 추가로 연장하여 보관하도록 하고 있다. 때로 의료기록은 환자 사망 후 수년이 지난 경우에도 쓰일 수 있다. 환경오염이나 산업재해로 사망한 경우 몇 년 후에도 조사 과정에서 환자의 과거 의료기록이 필요할 때도 있다.

3) 남용(Abuses)

외부에 환자기록의 번역, 또는 작성과 보관을 위임하게 되는 경우 환자의 기밀에 대한 규칙이 위반될 수도 있다. 의료기록의 위조는 중범죄에 속한다.

III. 의료 서류 번역

□ 환자 접수(Patient Sign-In Sheet)

□ 환자 정보(Patient Information): 환자의 모든 신상, 과거 병력, 건강상태(comprehensive review of patient's medical history and physical exam), 보험정보(insurance information) 등에 대한 내용이 들어 있다.

□ 환자 진료기록(Patient Medical Chart Notes) 및 그 외의 사항들

□ 환자동의서(Consents): 진찰 및 치료동의서, 환자 의료정보 사용동의서, 검사동의서, 수술동의서 등이 포함된다.

□ 안내문
건강검진 프로그램
위내시경 검사 안내문
PET-CT 검사 안내문

1. 환자접수(Patients Sign In Sheet)

환자가 진료장소에 도착하면 치료를 받기 위해 가장 먼저 등록을 하게 된다. 현재 대개의 종합병원이나 개인 병원에서는 도착을 구두로 알리고 번호표를 받아 진료 차례를 기다리게 되는데 이처럼 기록하여 등록을 하면 진료를 준비하는 데 도움이 된다.

1) Patients Sign In Sheet

(1) form A

일반적인 환자 등록 용지로 환자 이름과 진료 의사 이름, 도착 시간과 실재 약속 시간을 기록하여 순서대로 진료 받을 수 있도록 한다.

환자의 이름이나 그 외 정보가 노출되지 않도록 기록 후 스티커를 붙일 수 있도록 디자인된 것도 있다.

Patients Please Sign In

Date________________

	Patient's Name (Please Print)	Doctor's Name	Arriving Time	Appointment Time
1				
2				
3				
4				
5				
6				
7				
8				
9				
10				
11				
12				
13				
14				
15				
16				
17				
18				

(2) form B

환자정보의 보안을 위해 한 종이에 여러 명의 환자가 기록하지 않고 개인별로 등록하도록 만들어진 경우이다.

Patients Sign In

Patient Name: DOB:

New Patient? ☐ yes ☐ no

Date: Arrival Time:

Appointment for Doctor:

Please Note Changes in: ☐ address ☐ phone ☐ employment
☐ health insurance ☐ co-pay

Sign ______________________

단어 정리

☐ Patient Name	☐ 환자 이름
☐ DOB	☐ 생년월일(Date of Birth의 약어)
☐ New Patient?	☐ 처음 오시는 환자입니까?
☐ yes	☐ 네
☐ no	☐ 아니요
☐ Date	☐ 오늘 날짜
☐ Arrival Time	☐ 도착시간
☐ Appointment for Doctor	☐ 어느 의사에게 진료약속이 되어 있습니까?
☐ Please Note Changes in	☐ 개인정보의 변동이 있으면 표시해 주십시오
☐ address	☐ 주소
☐ phone	☐ 전화
☐ employment	☐ 직장
☐ health insurance	☐ 건강보험
☐ Sign	☐ 서명

2) Hospital Sign In Sheet

대학병원 혹은 입원, 진료, 검사 등이 종합적으로 이루어지는 병원에 진료를 위해 방문한 환자의 도착과 진료등록을 알리는 기록 용지의 예이다. 환자의 방문 내용을 상세히 기록하여 진료 준비를 하고 또 환자에 따라서 진료실까지 동행해 줄 보조원이 필요한 경우 이러한 서비스도 제공하도록 조처를 취할 수 있다.

여기에서도 환자의 정보 보안을 위해 기록 후 용지를 기록이 없는 쪽이 위로 가도록 하는 요청 내용이 있다.

미국과 같이 HIPAA라는 법적 보호를 요구하는 상황이 아니더라도 환자의 개인정보, 치료 내용 등은 항상 환자의 허락 없이는 누구에게도 유출되지 않도록 보호해 주는 것이 원칙이다.

Patient Sign In Sheet ①

PATIENT SIGN IN SHEET
WELCOME TO (NAME) HOSPITAL ADMITTING

Please fill out the information below and FLIP the sheet over for confidentiality. Thank you.

______________________	__________	____		
Patient Name(Please Print)	Date	□ Main	□ FOI	□ Main Admit

REASON FOR VISIT: (Please cheek one)

□ Ultrasound	□ Block	□ Coumadin Clinic
□ CT San	□ GI Lab	□ Cardiopulmonary
□ MRI	□ Specials	□ Direct Admit
□ PET Scan	□ Surgery	□ Nuclear
□ UGI	□ Lab	□ OBO
□ X-ray	□ Rahab Services	□ Other__________
□ Echo	□ Pre-Op	□ Financial Counselor

PLEASE DO NOT WRITE IN THIS AREA–ADMISSION STAFF USE ONEY

________________ Patient Appt Time		□ Express □ Quick □ Full	
________________ Patient Arrival Time	________________ Greeters Initials		
________________ Registration Start Time		________________ Escort Department Time	
________________ Registration End Time	________________ Registrars Initials	____________ Escort Drop Off Time	____________ Escort Initials

단어 정리

☐ PATIENT SIGN IN SHEET
환자가 병원에 도착하여 진료를 받기 위해 서명을 하는 용지

☐ WELCOME TO (NAME) HOSPITAL ADMITTING
저희 (병원이름)병원에 오신 것을 환영합니다

☐ Please fill out the information below and FLIP the sheet over for confidentiality. Thank you
아래 내용을 기록하시고 환자정보가 누설되지 않도록 용지를 뒤집어 놓으세요. 감사합니다

☐ sign in	☐ 서명하여 도착을 알게 하다(반대말: sign out)
☐ confidentiality	☐ 기밀성, 부적절한 누설방지
☐ Patient Name (Please Print)	☐ 환자 이름(영문이름인 경우 "Print" 하라는 것은 필기체로 기록하지 말고 대문자나 소문자를 써서 정자로 기록하라는 의미이다)
☐ Date	☐ 날짜
☐ Main	☐ Main Building을 뜻하며 병원 건물 내에 여러 가지 검사 및 치료를 받으러 온 경우를 말한다.
☐ FOI	☐ FOI란 Freedom of Information의 뜻으로 환자가 병원에 온 이유에 대해 기록하고 싶지 않을 때 여기에 표시하면 된다.
☐ Main Admit	☐ Main Admit란 치료가 아니라 접수부에 볼일이 있어서 병원에 온 경우(예를 들어 서류, 수납 등에 관계된 일 등)
☐ REASON FOR VISIT (Please check one)	☐ 방문의 이유(하나만 표시하세요)
☐ Ultrasound	☐ 초음파를 이용해 치료(진료)하는 일
☐ CT Scan	☐ 단층촬영. CAT Scan
☐ MRI	☐ 자기(磁氣)공명단층촬영장치[영상법] Magneticmagnetic Resonance Imager[Imaging]의 약어
☐ PET Scan	☐ PET 스캔, 양전자방사단층촬영에 의한 화상검사
☐ UGI	☐ 위장 상부위장조영술이란 의미로 조영제를 경구 투여한 후에 X선을 촬영해 위 점막 표면의 변화를 관찰한다. Upper Gastrointestinal의 약어
☐ X-ray	☐ X선 촬영
☐ Echo	☐ 초음파 심장 검진. Echocardiography의 약어
☐ Block	☐ regional anesthesia, 즉 부분적 마취를 의미한다. 예를 들어서 'ankle block'이란 무릎의 경골 신경주위에 마취 주사를 놓아 발

을 마비시키는 것(regional anesthesia of the foot by injection of anesthetic around the tibial nerves at the ankle)을 말한다.

- ☐ GI Lab — ☐ 위장에 관계된 검사실을 말한다. GI는 GastroIntestinal, Lab은 Laboratory의 약어
- ☐ Specials — ☐ 병원에서 일어나는 평상적 진료 외의 다른 진료들을 포함한다. 환자의 상황에 맞추어 어떤 특정 진료나 치료(Therapy)가 이루어질 경우를 말한다.
- ☐ Surgery — ☐ 수술을 받으러 온 경우
- ☐ Lab — ☐ 검사실 방문인 경우. Laboratory의 약어
- ☐ Rahab Services — ☐ 환자가 재활을 위한 치료를 받으러 병원에 온 경우이다. Rehab은 Rehabilitation의 약어
- ☐ Pre-Op — ☐ 수술 전에 선행되어야 할 모든 과정을 포함한다. Pre란 '-전(before)'이라는 의미이고 OP란 Operation(수술)의 약어
- ☐ Coumadin Clinic — ☐ Coumadin이란 약은 피를 묽게 하는 항응고제(anticoagulant)인데 혈액에 혈전의 증세를 보이는 환자들이 상담을 통해서 복용하는 약이다. 즉, 이 약과 관련된 진료를 하는 곳이다.
- ☐ Cardiopulmonary — ☐ 심폐기능 진료소. Cardio(Cardiology)는 심장, pulmonary는 폐에 관계되는 치료
- ☐ Direct Admit — ☐ Admit는 Admission(입원)을 의미하며 입원을 위해 내원한 경우
- ☐ Other__________ — ☐ 그 외의 다른 이유가 있어서 내원한 경우 여기에 표시하고 옆에 그 이유를 기입하면 된다.

☞ 환자가 기록하지 않는 내용

PLEASE DO NOT WRITE IN THIS AREA–ADMISSION STAFF USE ONEY			
Patient Appt. Time		☐ Express	
Patient Arrival Time	Greeters Initials		
Registration Start Time			
Registration End Time	Registrars Initials	Escort Drop Off Time	Escort Initials

환자에게 기입을 요구하는 내용 외에 병원에서 직접 의료진이나 직원이 기입해야 할 내용이 있을 때 대개는 금방 구별되도록 내용을 네모 안에 넣어 놓는다.

단어 정리

- ☐ PLEASE DO NOT WRITE IN THIS AREA-ADMISSION STAFF USE ONLY — ☐ 이 부분은 기입하지 마세요－접수처 직원만 이 기입가능
- ☐ Patient Appt. Time — ☐ 환자의 (진료)예약 시간
  Appt는 Appointment(예약)의 약어
- ☐ Patient Arrival Time — ☐ 환자가 병원에 도착한 시간
- ☐ Greeters Initials — ☐ 접수인 이름(Initial이란 이름 전체가 아니라 이름 일부를 간단히 쓰면 된다)
- ☐ Registiration Start Time — ☐ 접수를 시작한 시간
- ☐ Registration End Time — ☐ 접수를 끝낸 시간
- ☐ Registrars Initials — ☐ 접수 직원 이름 기입
- ☐ Express — ☐ 급하게 치료를 해야 할 경우
- ☐ Escort Drop Off Time — ☐ 환자를 직원이 동반해서 데리고 갈 경우 진료장소에 도착한 시간 기입
- ☐ Escort Initials — ☐ 동반한 직원 이름 기입

2. 환자정보(Patient Information) 및 환자문진표(Patient Questionnaire)

Patient Information ① 한글본

환자 정보

×××××× ××× MD ○○○ Medical Clinic
##구 ##동 #### (02) ×××－××××

1. 본인신상정보

이름(영) ______ (한) ______
주소 ______
______
성별 남 여 나이 ____ 생년월일 ______
미혼 기혼 사별 별거 이혼
소셜 시큐러티# ___ ______
직업 ______
근무처 ______
직장 주소 ______
직장 전화번호 ______
배우자 이름 ______
생년월일 ______ SS# ______
직업 ______
근무처 ______

2. 보험

주 가입자 이름 ______
환자와의 관계 ______
생년월일 ______ SS# ______
보험회사 이름 ______
Group# ______
2차 보험이 있습니까? □네 □아니오
2차 보험 주(主)가입자 이름 ______
생년월일 ______ SS# ______
보험회사 이름 ______
Group# ______

위임 및 의료기록 제공에 대한 동의

본인(혹은 왼쪽 난에 기재한 환자)은 위에 밝힌 대로 보험에 가입하고 있음을 확인하며, 보험 회사가 진료와 관련된 비용을 Dr. Dennis Kim에게 지불하도록 허락합니다. 또한 보험에서 지급되지 않은 잔여 치료비에 대해서는 본인 자신이 부담할 책임이 있음을 확인합니다. 또한 의사가 보험료 지불을 위해 보험 회사에 본인의 건강/질병에 관한 기록을 제공하는 것을 허락합니다. 위의 모든 사실을 다음의 서명으로 확인합니다.

______
보험 주(主)가입자 서명

______ ______
환자와의 관계 날짜

3. 전화번호

자택 ______ 직장 ______ ext ______
연락하기 가장 좋은 시간/장소 ______

비상시 연락처
이름 ______ 관계 ______
전화번호 ______

4. 가족 병력기록

오늘 클리닉에 오신 주된 이유는 무엇입니까? ______
이전 주치의 이름 ______ 전화번호와 주소 ______
______
최근에 보신(혹은 현재 보시는)의사/전문의 이름을 모두 적어 주십시오 ______
______

가족 병력

아버지 생존 사망 병력 ____________ 사망연령 ________ 사망원인 ________

어머니 생존 사망 병력 ____________ 사망연령 ________ 사망원인 ________

형제자매 생존자 수 ________ 사망자 수 ________ 사망연령 ________ 사망원인 ________

형제자매들의 병력 ____________________________

자녀들 생존자 수 ________ 사망자 수 ________ 사망연령 ________ 사망원인 ________

형제자매들의 병력 ____________________________

다음 중 혈연이 있는 친족들에게 있는 질병에 O표 하십시오. 당뇨, 심장병, 고혈압, 천식, 혈액병, 암(무슨 암?   ), 중풍, 신장병, 알코올 혹은 약물중독, 알레르기, 우울증, 불안/초조 관절염, 갑상선 질환, 기타:

5 건강/병력 기록 다음의 모든 정보는 비밀이 보장됩니다.

지금 혹은 지난 1년 동안 느끼신 증상들에 체크하십시오.

일반

( ) 신열/오한
( ) 두통
( ) 우울/불안 초조
( ) 어지러움/현기증
( ) 불면
( ) 식욕감퇴
( ) 체중 증가/감소
( ) 병원 입원

근육 골격

약하거나 통증이 있으면 체크

( ) 팔 ( ) 골반
( ) 허리 ( ) 다리
( ) 발 ( ) 목
( ) 손 ( ) 어깨

비뇨기

( ) 소변에 피가 나온다
( ) 소변을 자주 본다
( ) 소변 조절이 안 된다
( ) 소변 볼 때 아프다

소화기

( ) 메스꺼움
( ) 구토
( ) 복통
( ) 변비
( ) 설사
( ) 변에 피가 나온다
( ) 변 색깔이 검다
( ) 황달
( ) 음식 삼키기가 힘들다
( ) 트림이 잦다

심장 혈관

( ) 가슴에 통증
( ) 고혈압
( ) 부정맥
( ) 발/발목이 붓는다
( ) 숨이 가쁘다
( ) 걸을 때 종아리가 아프다
( ) 기절
( ) 저혈압

눈/귀/코/목

( ) 눈이 침침하다
( ) 사물이 둘로 보인다
( ) 귀가 아프다
( ) 청력 감퇴
( ) 계절 알레르기
( ) 목이 아프다
( ) 목소리가 변한다
( ) 코피
( ) 이명(귀울림)
( ) 축농증
( ) 잦은 기침
( ) 입이 마르다
( ) 구취
( ) 잇몸 출혈

피부

( ) 멍이 잘 든다
( ) 두드러기
( ) 가려움
( ) 점(點)색깔/크기가 변한다

남성에 한함

( ) 발기 부전
( ) 고환이 붓거나 종양
( ) 음경 출투
( ) 소변 줄기가 약하다
( ) 국부 통증

여성에 한함

( ) 팹 검사 이상
( ) 주기 외(外) 출혈
( ) 유방에 이상
( ) 이상 질분비(냉)
( ) 국부 통증
( ) 임신

마지막 월경 주기가 언제?
____

마지막 팹 검사?
____

마지막 유방암 X-ray?
____

지금 가지고 있거나 과거에 있었던 병력에 체크하십시오.

( ) AIDS	( ) 신장병	( ) 고혈압
( ) 맹장염	( ) 당뇨	( ) 췌장암
( ) 관절염	( ) 천식	( ) 암
( ) 천식	( ) 간질	( ) 편두통
( ) 혈액병	( ) 녹내장	( ) 결핵
( ) 갱년기	( ) 심장병	( ) 갑상선질환
( ) 백내장	( ) 간염	( ) 전립선질환
( ) 담석증	( ) 허피스	( ) 위궤양
( ) 알콜/약물중독 기타	( ) 콜레스테롤	( ) 성병

수술 받으신 것/연도
____
____
____

상해(傷害)/연도
____
____
____

수혈 받으신 적 있습니까?
없다 있다 언제?

<table>
<tr><th>6. 약(藥)/알레르기</th><th>7. 건강습관</th></tr>
<tr><td>지금 드시고 있는 모든 약을 다 쓰십시오.
____
____
____
____
약 알레르기(부작용)? ______________
기타 알레르기? ______________</td><td>흡연 아니오____ 네____ 하루 몇 갑? ________
음주 아니오____ 네____ 일주일에 몇 번? ______
다른 약물 ______________
카페인 커피/콜라 하루 몇 잔? ______________
운동 일주일에 몇 번? __________
한 번에 몇 분씩? ____________
물을 하루에 몇 잔 마십니까? ______________
유해물질에 노출되어 있습니까? 아니오___ 네___
식사 규칙적 불규칙적 육식( )% 채식( )%
하루 몇 끼? ______ 간식? _______ 밤참? ______</td></tr>
<tr><th colspan="2">8. 서명</th></tr>
<tr><td colspan="2">본인은 위에 기재한 내용들이 사실이며, 또한 이 양식을 작성함에 있어서 본인이 빠뜨린 항목에 대해서 의사나 클리닉의 책임이 없음을 확인합니다.
서명 ______________________ 날짜 ______________________
검토자 서명 ______________________ 날짜 ______________________</td></tr>
</table>

Patient Information ① 영문본

Patient Infomation

××××××× ××× MD ○○○ Medical Clinic
(02) ×××－××××

1. PATIENT INFOMATION

Name ______________________
Address______________________
Sex M F Age________ Birthdate_________
single married widowed separated divorced
Social Security# ______________________
Occupation ______________________
Employer ______________________
Employer Address ______________________
Employer Phone ______________________
Spouse's Name ______________________
Birthdate ____________ SS# ____________
Occupation ______________________
Employer ______________________

2. INSURANCE

Who's responsible to this Account? ____________
Relationship to Patient ______________________
Birthdate ______________ SS# ____________
Insurance Co ______________________
Group # ______________________
Is Patient Covered by Additional Insurance?
☐ Yes ☐ No
Subscriber Name ______________________
Birthdate ______________ SS# ____________
Insurance Co ______________________
Group # ______________________

Assignment and Release

I, Undersigned, certify that I(or my dependent)has insurance coverage as above, and assign directly to Dr, Dennis Kim all insurance benefits. If any, otherwise payable to me for service rendered, I understand that I am financially responsible for all charges whether or not paid by insurance, I hereby authorize the doctor to release all information necessary to secure the payment of benefits, I authorize the use of this signature on all insurance submissions.

____
Responsible Party Signature

______________ ______________
Relationship Date

3. PHONE NUMBERS

Home __________ Work __________ ext __________
Best time and place to reach you ____________
IN CASE OF EMERGENCY, CONTACT
Name ______________ Relationship ____________
Phone# ______________________

4. FAMILY MEDICAL HISTORY

What is the reason for our visit today? ______________________
Who was your primary care physician before? ______________ Phone#Address ______________
____
List al physicians/specialists you are seeing or have seen recently ______________________

FAMILY MEDICAL HISTORY
Father Alive? Y N Diseases ______________ Age of Death ________ Cause of Death __________
Mother Alive? Y N Diseases ______________ Age of Death ________ Cause of Death __________
Siblings No. Alive _________No. Deceased ________ Age of Death ________ Cause of Death __________
Diseases of Siblings ____

Children No. Alive _________ No. Deceased ________ Age of Death _________ Cause of Death ________

Diseases of Siblings ____

CIRCLE ILLNESSES WHICH HAVE OCCURRED IN YOUR BLOOD RELATIVES Diabetes, Heart Disease, Cancer(What Type?), High Blood Pressure, Stroke, Alcoholism, Asthma, Allergy Mental Illness(What type?)

Other:

5 MEDICAL HISTORY All information is strictly confidential

Check Symptoms you have or have had past on year

GENERAL	GASTROINTESTINAL	EENT	MEN ONLY
( ) Fever/Chills	( ) Nausea	( ) Bharry Vision	( ) Erection Difficulties
( ) Headache	( ) Vomiting	( ) Double Vision	( ) Lump in testicles
( ) Depression/Nervousness	( ) Abdominal Pain	( ) Ear Pain	( ) Penile Discharge
( ) Dizziness/Fainting	( ) Constipation	( ) Hearing Difficulties	( ) Weak Urine Stream
( ) Loss of Sleep	( ) Diarrhea	( ) Hay Fever	( ) Penile Pain
( ) Loss of Appetite	( ) Blood in Stool	( ) Sore Throat	
( ) Weight Loss/Gain	( ) Black stool	( ) Change of Voice	WOMEN ONLY
( ) Hospital Admission	( ) Jaundice	( ) Nosebleed	( ) Abnormal Pap Smear
MUSCULOSKELETAL	( ) Difficulty Swallowing	( ) Ringing in the Ear	( ) Abnormal Bleeding
Pain weakness numbness in:	( ) Belching	( ) Sinus Problems	( ) Severe Menstrual Pain
( ) Arms ( ) Hips		( ) Limp in the Neck	( ) Hot Flashes
( ) Back ( ) Legs	CARDIOVASCULAR	( ) Dry Mouth	( ) Nipple Discharge
( ) Feet ( ) Neck	( ) Chest Pain	( ) Halitosis(Bad Breath)	( ) Vaginal Discharge
( ) Hands ( ) Shoulders	( ) High Blood Pressure	( ) Bleeding Gums	( ) Pelvic Pain
GENITOURINARY	( ) Irregular Heart Beat		Date of Last Menstruation
	( ) Feet/Ankle Swelling	SKIN	________________
( ) Blood in Urine	( ) Shortness of Breath	( ) Bruises Easily	Date of Last Pap Smear:
( ) Frequent Urination	( ) Leg Pain in Walking	( ) Hives	________________
( ) Lack of Bladder Control	( ) Pressing Out	( ) Itching	Date of Last Mammogram
( ) Painful Urination	( ) Low Blood Pressure	( ) Change in Moles	________________

Check conditions you have or have had

( ) AIDS	( ) Kidney Disease	( ) High Blood Pressure
( ) Appendicitis	( ) Diabetes	( ) Liver Disease
( ) Arthritis	( ) Emphysema	( ) Pancreatitis
( ) Asthma	( ) Epilepsy	( ) Migraine
( ) Bleeding Disorders	( ) Glaucoma	( ) Cancer
( ) Breast Lump	( ) Heart Disease	( ) Thyroid Disease
( ) Cataracts	( ) Hepatitis	( ) Prostate Disease
( ) Gallstones	( ) Herpes	( ) Ulcer
( ) Substance Abuse	( ) High Cholesterol	( ) Veneral Disease

Operations/Year

____

____

____

Significant Injuries/Year

____

____

____

Blood Transfusion? N Y When?

6. MEDICATIONS/ALLERGIES	7. HEALTH HABITS
List All the Medications You are Taking ________________________ ________________________ ________________________ ________________________ Drug Allergies? ________________ Other Allergies? ________________	Cigarette Smoking: N Y ____ packs per day(Quit? When?) Alcohol: N Y ______ drinks per week(Quit? When?) Other Drugs ________________ Caffeine ________ cups of ________ per day Exercise _____ times a week _____ min each time What type of Exercise? ____________ Drinking Water ________ cups per day Exposed to Hazardous Substances? N Y _______

8. SIGNATURES
I certify tat the above information is correct to the best of my knowledge. I will not bold my doctor or my members of his staff responsible for errors or omissions that I may have made in the completion of this form. Signature ____________________ Date ____________________ Reviewed by ____________________ Date ____________________

Patient Information ② 한글본

비뇨기과 환자병력 양식

오늘 날짜_______________ 건강검진 날짜_______________
성_______________ 이름_______________ M.I. __________
사회보장번호_______________ 생년월일____________________
키_____________ 몸무게_______________

주요문제(오늘 병원을 방문하신 가장 중요한 이유는 무엇입니까?)

____
____
____
____

아픈 곳: 복부 등 다리 그 외____________________

1에서 10까지의 수로 통증을 표현할 때 10이 가장 통증이 심한 경우를 말한다면 당신의 통증은 어떤 수로 표현할 수 있습니까? 1, 2, 3, 4, 5, 6, 7, 8, 9, 10

언제 처음 문제를 알게 되었나요? 이틀 전, 이주 전, 한달 전, 그 외__________

어떤 경우 도움이 되거나 혹은 통증이 더 악화됩니까? 움직일 때, 일어서 있을 때, 그 외__________

얼마나 오래 문제(통증)가 지속됩니까? 30분, 1시간, 항상, 그 외____________________

(문제가 있을 때) 동시에 일어나는 다른 문제가 있습니까? 아니오____ 네____ 있다면 설명하시오.

문제가(통증이) 지속적입니까 혹은 변합니까? 약하다가 심해진다___항상 있다___그 외____

문제가 정상 생활에 방해가 됩니까? 아니오_____네_______ 있다면 설명하시오.

습관성 중독:

흡연? 네______아니오__________얼마나 오래 되었고 얼마나 많이 피나요?____________________
알코올 소비? 전혀 안함_______별로 안함_______가끔________중간 정도_______자주_______

약과 음식 알레르기:

약	반응상태	시기(대략)

다음 페이지 넘겨 완성하시오

Page 1

병력기록지 계속

현재 복용하고 계신 약
(비타민과 천연약재 포함)

약명 강도 하루 복용치 얼마나 오래 복용하고 있나

____
____
____
____
____
____

수술과 대략의 수술 시기를 기입하세요:

____
____
____
____
____
____

과거 병력과 대략의 시기를 기입해 주세요:

____
____
____
____
____
____

환자 서명 ______________________________

의사만 기록(의견/메모)

의사 서명 ______________________________

Page 2

Patient Information ② 영문본

UROLOGY PATIENT HISTORY FORM

Today's Date__________________ Date of Last Physical Exam____________________

Last Name___________________First Name__________________M.I.______________

Social Security No.__________________Date of Birth__________________________

Height________________Weight____________________

CHIEF COMPLAINT(What is the main reason for your visit today?)

____

____

____

____

Location of the problem: Abdomen Back Leg Other_______________________

On a scale of 1-10, with 10 being the most severe, circle the number that best describe the problem.
1 2 3 4 5 6 7 8 9 10

When did you first notice the problem? 2days ago, 2weeks ago, 1month ago, Other____________

Does anything help or make the problem worse? Moving around, Standing up, Other____________

How long does the problem last? 30min, 1hr, It's always there, Other___________________________

Is anything else occurring at the same time? No_____Yes__________If yes, please explain

Is the problem constant or variable? Dull then Sharp Always there Other______________________

Dose the problem interfere with your normal functions? No_____Yes________If yes, please explain

HABITS:

Smoke? Yes_______No____________If yes, how long and how much____________________________

Alcohol Consumption? No________Rare________Occasional_________Moderate________Often________

DRUG and FOOD ALLERGIES:

DRUG ____________ Type of Reaction ____________ When(approximately)

____

____

____

____

____

PLEASE TURN OVER TO COMPLETE

Page 1

MEDICAL HISTORY FORM CONTINUED

PLEASE ANY MEDICATIONS YOU ARE CURRENTLY TAKING

(include Vitamins and Herbs)

Medication Name	Strength	Amount taken daily	How long using

Please list surgeries and approximately when they occurred:

____
____
____
____
____
____

Please list major illnesses and approximate time of their occuring:

____
____
____
____
____
____

Patinets Signature______________________________

Physicians use only(comments/note):

Physicians Signature ______________________________

Page 2

Patient Information ③ 한글본

병원 주소

환자정보

저희 병원에 오신 것을 환영합니다. 이 내용은 환자를 진료하는 데 의사에게 귀중한 자료입니다. 가능한 자세하게 빠진 것 없이 기록해 주십시오.

개인정보

이름: ______________________ 주소: ______________________
도시명: ______________________ 주: ____________우편번호: __________
집전화: ____________ 생년월일 ___/___/___ 나이: _____ 성별: 남 여
직장: ____________ 직장전화: ____________ 사회보장번호: ___-___-___
업무 종류: ______________________________
혼인 여부: ___ M ___ S ___ W ___ D 배우자 이름: ______________
비상연락처: ______________________________
주치의: ______________________________
누가 저희 병원을 추천했나요? ______________________
이메일 주소: ______________________________

현재 건강 상태

주된 혹은 일차적인 문제점:
____
____
문제가 얼마나 심각한가요? _______ 경 _______ 중 _______ 심각
이전에 발병했던 병인가요? ___네 ___ 아니오
이 상태가 언제 시작되었나요? ______________________
이 문제로 만났던 다른 의사가 있나요? ______________
이전에 만난 의사의 소견/진단명: ______________________
이 상태가: _________ 직업과 관계가 있다 __________ 자동차와 관계가 있다 _________ 부상과 관계가 있다 그 외: ______________
이 문제 외의 다른 혹은 부차적인 문제: ______________________
다른 건강문제: ______ 네 ______ 아니오 '네'이면 어떤 문제인지 설명해 주십시오: ____________
현재 복용하고 계신 마약이나 일반약
___ 진통제/근육 이완제 ___ 혈압약 ___ 위장약
___ 진정제 ___ 항생제 그 외: ________

과거 병력

주요 수술(부위): ___ 머리 ___ 목/목구멍 ___ 가슴/심장/폐 ___ 등 ___ 복부 그 외: ______
골절이 있었습니까? ___네 ___ 아니오 무슨 골절이었습니까? ______________
예전에 낙상 혹은 사고 경력이 있습니까? ___ 네 ___ 아니오 언제입니까? ____________
예전에 입원경력이 있습니까? ___ 네 ___ 아니오 왜 입원했습니까? ______________
이전의 척추교정지압 치료경험이 있습니까? ___ 네 ___ 아니오 치료의: ______________
가족 중에 비슷한 병을 앓은 분이 있습니까? ___ 네 ___ 아니오
같이 일하는 사람 중 비슷한 병을 앓은 분이 있습니까? ___ 네 ___ 아니오
어떤 스포츠나 운동 프로그램에 참여하고 계십니까? ___ 네 ___ 아니오

다음 페이지 넘겨 완성하시오

Page 1

아래에 열거된 질병과 기능장애들은 병원을 찾으신 이유와는 무관할지도 모릅니다. 그러나 이와 같은 정보는 우리의 치료와 병에 접근하는 데 있어 환자에게 일어날 반응에 영향을 끼칠 수도 있습니다.

해당되는 질병을 표시해 주세요

___소아마비
___당뇨
___암
___그 외:___________
___심장병
___만성피로

___관절염
___간질
___에이즈 혹은 에이즈 관련 증세
___입담배
___잦은 질병
___알레르기

섭취 및 사용
___알코올
___마약
___진통제
___처방약

지난 6개월 동안 앓았던 적이 있는 문제(질환)에 표시해 주세요

근골계
___요통
___어깨 사이의 통증
___목(근육)의 통증
___팔의 통증
___관절통/뻣뻣함
___보행에 장애
___씹는 데 장애 - 턱관절장애
___일반적 뻣뻣함

순환기 호흡
___가슴 통증
___숨가쁨
___혈압
___불규칙적인 심장박동
___심장 문제
___폐의 문제
___뇌졸중

눈-귀-코-목
___시각적 방해들
___치과적 문제
___목아픔
___이(귀)통
___청각장애
___코막힘
___공동분비물
___통증-이마 혹은 얼굴

신경계

신경계
___두통
___불안감
___마비/저림
___근육 무력
___어지러움
___건망증
___우울
___기절
___발작/간질
___냉한 수족
___스트레스
___흔들림/떨림

소화-배설
___입맛 없음
___과도한 갈증
___잦은 구역질
___설사
___변비
___치질
___체중감소/증가
___가스/더부룩함
___속쓰림
___대변의 변화

비뇨기-생식기
___소변 시 통증
___아주 드문 소변
___잦은 소변
___소변줄기가 약함
___방광 조절 능력의 상실
___생식기 통증

여성에게만 해당
___생리통/생리불순
___생리시 요통
___유방에 통증/혹(덩어리)
임신중입니까? __네 __아니오
__확실하지 않음

아픈 부위에 표시하십시오:

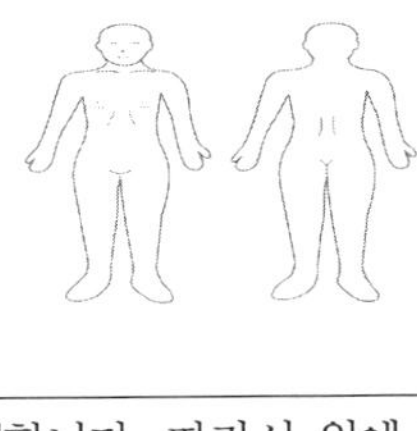

(×)통증 (○)경련 (•)마비

저는 치료가 의사선생님께서 아시는 바에 의해 결정된다는 것을 이해합니다. 따라서 위에 제가 기록한 내용들은 제가 아는 한 정직하고 완전하게 기록되었습니다. 또한 저는 치료란 의사가 결과에 대해 책임질 수 있는 정확한 과학이 아니며 내가 의존할 수 있는 것이 아닌 것을 이해합니다. 저는 의사의 전문가적 의견은 어떤 증세에 대한 진단가 치료에 대한 책임에 있다는 것 또한 이해합니다.

환자 서명_______________________ **날짜**______________________

Page 2

Patient Information Sheet ③ 영문본

Hospital address

PATIENT INFORMATION

Welcome to our practice. Please answer the following questions. This will give the doctor valuable information needed to help you. Please be as accurate and complete as possible.

PERSONAL INFORMATION

Name: ______________________ Address: ______________________
City: ______________________ State: ____________ Zip: ____________
Home Phone: ______________________ Date of Birth ___/___/___ Age: _____ Sex: M F
Business/Employer: ______________ Work Phone: ______________ SSN: ___-___-___
Type of Work Performed: ______________________________
Marital Status: ___ M ___ S ___ W ___ D Spouse's Name: ______________________
In Case of Emergency Notify: ______________________________
Name of Family Physician: ______________________________
Who referred you to our office? ______________________________
E-mail address: ______________________________

CURRENT HEALTH CONDITION

Main or Primary Complaint:
____
____
How Severe is This Problem: ___ Mild ___ Moderate ___ Severe
Previous Occurrences: ___ Yes ___ No
When Did This Condition Begin: ______________________________
Other Doctors Seen For this Complaint: ______________________
Previous Doctor's Opinion/Diagnosis: ______________________
Is Condition: ___ Job Related ___ Auto Related ___ Injury Other: ______________
Other or Secondary Complaints: ______________________________
Other Health Problems: ___Yes ___ No If "Yes", please describe: ______________
Drugs or Medicines Now Taking:
___ Pain Killers/Muscle Relaxers ___ Blood Pressure Medicine ___ Stomach Medicine
___ Tranquilizers ___ Antibiotics Other: ________

PAST HEALTH HISTORY

Major Surgeries: ___ Head ___ Neck/Throat ___ Chest/Heart/Lung ___ Back ___ Abdominal Other: _____
Previous Fractures: ___ Yes ___ No What: ______________________
Previous Falls or Accidents: ___ Yes ___ No When: ______________
Previous Hospitalization: ___ Yes ___ No Why: ______________
Previous Chiropractic Care: ___ Yes ___ No Doctor: ______________
Has Anyone Else In Your Family Had A Similar Problem? ___ Yes ___ No
Has Anyone With Whom You've Worked Had A Similar Problem? ___ Yes ___ No
Do You Participate In Any Sports or Exercise Programs? ___ Yes ___ No

PLEASE TURN OVER TO COMPLETE

Page 1

Below is a list of disease and disorders that may seem unrelated to the purpose of your appointment. However, the following information may affect your response to our care as well as our approach to handling your case. Please complete the following as carefully as possible.

Check any of the following that applies to you

___Polio
___Diabetes
___Cancer
___Other:____________
___Heart Disease
___Chronic Fatigue

___Arthritis
___Epilepsy
___AIDS or ARC
___Tobacco
___Frequent Illnesses
___Allergies

INTAKE OR USE
___Alcohol
___Recreational Drugs
___Pain Relievers
___Prescribed Drugs

Check any problem that you have had in the past 6 months:

Muscles-Skeleton
___Low Back Pain
___Pain Between Shoulders
___Neck Pain
___Arm Pain
___Joint Pain/Stiffness
___Problems Walking
___Difficulty Chewing - TMJ (Temporo Mandibular Joint)
___General Stiffness

Circulation-Breathing
___Chest Pain
___Shortness of Breath
___Blood Pressure Problems
___Irregular Heart Rate
___Heart Problems
___Lung Problems
___Stroke

Eye-Ear-Nose-Throat
___Visual Disturbances
___Dental Problems
___Sore Throat
___Ear Aches
___Difficulty Hearing
___Stuffy Nose
___Sinus Drainage/Pain
___Pain - Forehead or Face

Nerve System

Nerve System
___Headaches
___Nervousness
___Numbness/Tingling
___Muscular Weakness
___Dizziness
___Forgetfulness
___Depression
___Fainting
___Convulsions/Seizures
___Cold Hands Feet
___Stress
___Shaking/Tremors

Digestion-Elimination
___Poor Appetite
___Excessive Thirst
___Frequent Nausea
___Diarrhea
___Constipation
___Hemorrhoids
___Weight Loss/Gain
___Gas/Bloating
___Heartburn
___Change in Stools

Urinary-Genitals
___Pain with Urination
___Infrequent Urination
___Frequent Urination
___Weak Urine Stream
___Loss Of Bladder Control
___Pain in Genitals

Female Only
___Menstrual Pain/Irregularity
___Low Back Pain w/Periods
___Breast Pain/Lumps
Are you Pregnant? __Yes __No __Not Sure

Please mark your areas of complaint:

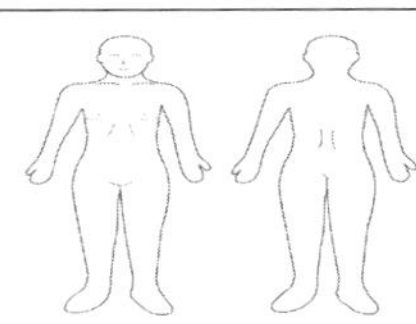

(×)Pain (○)Spasm (•)Numb

I understand that my care in this office may involve the making of judgments that are based upon the facts known by the doctor. Therefore, the above information is true and complete to the best of my knowledge. I also understand that a doctor practicing any healing art which neither guarantee results nor should rely upon for results because it is an inexact science. I further understand that the doctor's professional expertise lies in responsible for the diagnosis or treatment of any medical condition.

Patient
Signature________________________ Date ______________________

Page 2

Patient Infomation ④ 한글본

병원 이름

환자 번호 ____________________ 날짜 ___ / ___ / ___

성 ____________________ 이름 ____________________ 생년월일 ________ 나이 ___

병원에 보낸 의사 ____ 성별 □여성 □ 남성

집전화 ________________________________ 직장전화 _________×___________

연락하기 좋은 시간: ____________________

정기 검사 입니까? □네 □아니오

마지막 유방암 검사는 언제 어디서 하셨습니까? ____________________________

개인 위험 요소

	나이	나이	
□**유전성 유방암**		□**병력** _____	
□유방1	□**유방암 경력**____	□유관이상과 형성	□유관악성종양
□유방2	□**난소암 경력**____	□소엽이상과 형성	□소엽악성종양

가족유방암 병력

친척	나이	폐경		나이	폐경
□어머니	________	□	□숙모	________	□
□자매	________	□	□할머니	________	□

부인과 병력

초경 나이 _______

폐경 나이 _______

첫 임신 나이 _______

유방재건

□오른쪽 날짜______	□실리콘 젤	□식염수
□왼쪽 날짜_______	□실리콘 젤	□식염수

개인 위험 요소들

	현재사용	사용기간
경구피임약	□	____년
에스트로겐	□	____년
프로게스테론	□	____년
타목시펜	□	____년
라록시판	□	____년
그 외 호르몬	□	____년

유방재건

유방수술 및 치료 내력

(날짜, 종류, 결과포함)

□유방조직검사 □유방종양절재 □유방절재

□낭종흡인술 □교정 □그 외

암 발견: □네 □아니오

____

____

____

유방암 진찰을 통해 유방진단과 마모그라피에서 발견할 수 없는 암을 찾기도 합니다.

□네 □아니오 주치의에게 유방암 진찰을 받으셨습니까?

환자 서명 ____________________ 날짜 _____ / ______ / _____

Patient Infomation ④ 영문본

Hospital Name

Patient ID ____________________ Date ___/___/___

Last _________________________ First ____________________ DOB _________ Age ____

Referred by ____ Sex ☐Female ☐Male

Home phone __________________________ Work phone _________×___________

Best Time to Contact: __________________

Is this a routine screening exam? ☐Yes ☐No

When and Where was your last mammogram? ________________________________

Personal Risk Factors

		at Age		at Age
☐Breast cancer gene			☐History of high-risk lesion ______	
☐BRCA1	☐History of breast cancer _____		☐Alypical ductal hyperplasia	☐ductal carcinoma in situ
☐BRCA2	☐History of ovarian cancer ____		☐Alypical lobular hyperplasia	☐lobular carcinoma in situ

Family History of Breast Cancer

Relative	at Age	Pre-menopause		at Age	Pre-menopause
☐Mother	__________	☐	☐Aunt	__________	☐
☐Sister	__________	☐	☐Grandmother	__________	☐

Gynecological History

First menstrual period at age _______

Menopause age _______

First full-term pregnancy at age _______

Breast Implants

☐Right Date________ ☐Silicone Gel ☐Saline

☐Left Date________ ☐Silicone Gel ☐Saline

Personal Risk Factors

	Currently Using	Dration of use
Oral Contraceptives	☐	____yrs
Estrogen	☐	____yrs
Progesterone	☐	____yrs
Tamoxifen	☐	____yrs
Raloxifene	☐	____yrs
Unspecified hormones	☐	____yrs

Breast Implants

Breast Surgical and Treatment History

(Inclued date, type, and result)

☐Breast Biopsy ☐Lumpectomy ☐Mastectomy

☐Cyst Aspiration ☐Reduction ☐Other:

Cancer Found: ☐Yes ☐No

A clinical breast exam is a very important part of breast evaluation and can identify cancers that are not able to be identified on mammography.

☐I have ☐have not had a clinical breast exam by my referring provider.

Patient Signature ____________________________ Date ______/_______/______

Patient Information ⑤ 한글본

환자 병력 및 섭취에 대한 질문서

기입방법: 첫 장은 방문 때마다 작성해 주세요

날짜 ______________________

작성하시는 데 도움이 필요하시면 저희 직원에게 요청하시기 바랍니다. 아시는 한 자세히 기입해 주세요. 아래 기입된 모든 건강 문제들을 입원 진료 중에 다 도와드리지는 못하지만 기입하신 내용을 통해 자녀분의 치료를 더욱 효과적으로 할 수 있습니다.

기록자 성함:______________ 어린이와의 관계:______________

현재 건강상태

왜 오늘 병원을 방문하셨습니까? ____________________________

☐ **우리 아이는 아래 표시한 내용 외에 다른 증세는 없습니다**

현재 자녀분의 증세나 상태에 해당하는 것에 표시해 주십시오

	기간		기간		기간
허약/피곤 ☐	________	시각장애 ☐	________	체중증가가 어려움 ☐	________
열/오한 ☐	________	쉰 목소리 ☐	________	체중 감소 ☐	________
간질 ☐	________	호흡장애 ☐	________	부족한 음식/음료 섭취 ☐	________
불면 ☐	________	쌕쌕거림 ☐	________	과다한 음식/음료 섭취 ☐	________
과다수면 ☐	________	기침 ☐	________	배뇨통 ☐	________
코골이 ☐	________	가슴통증 ☐	________	배뇨 횟수의 증가 ☐	________
두통 ☐	________	빠른 심장박동 ☐	________	혈뇨 ☐	________
귀/목(후비강)통증 ☐	________	심잡음 ☐	________	불규칙한/통증이 있는 생리 ☐	________
삼키기/씹기 불편함 ☐	________	위통 ☐	________	질의 분비물 ☐	________
목통증/부종 ☐	________	변비 ☐	________	관절/다리/팔통증 ☐	________
콧물 흘림 ☐	________	구토 ☐	________	쉽게 멍듦 ☐	________
눈 분비물/충혈 ☐	________	설사 ☐	________	노란색 피부/황달 ☐	________
청각장애 ☐	________	혈변 ☐	________	발진/피부 문제 ☐	________

☐그 외________

* 초진 환자나 예전과 다르게 변한 사항이 있으신 분은 다음 장을 기록하십시오.

병원 이름	

Patient History and Intake Form

DIRECTIONS: PLEASE FILL OUT THE FRONT PAGE AT EVERY VISIT

Date ____________________

If you need help completing this form please ask a staff member for help. Give as many details as you know. Please note that while we may not be able to address all of the health problems list on this sheet during this clinic visit, our knowledge of them may help us deal with your child's needs more effectively.

Your name: ______________ Your relationship to child: ______________

CURRENT HEALTH CONCERNS

Why are we seeing your child today? ______________________________

☐ My child has no other symptoms unless checked below

PLACE A CHECKMARK NEXT TO ANY SYMPTOM OR CONDITION YOUR CHILD CURRENTLY HAS

	How Long		How Long		How Long
Weakness/Tired ☐	______	Trouble Seeing ☐	______	Difficulty Gaining Weight ☐	______
Fever/Chills ☐	______	Hoarse Voice ☐	______	Weight Loss ☐	______
Seizures ☐	______	Trouble Breathing ☐	______	Poor Eating/Drinking ☐	______
Trouble Sleeping ☐	______	Wheeze ☐	______	Eats/Drinks Too Much ☐	______
Sleeps Too Much ☐	______	Cough ☐	______	Pain With Urination ☐	______
Snoring ☐	______	Chest Pain ☐	______	Increased Urination ☐	______
Headache ☐	______	Rapid Heart Rate ☐	______	Blood in Urine ☐	______
Ear/Throat Pain ☐	______	Heart Murmur ☐	______	Irregular/Painful Periods ☐	______
Trouble Swallowing/Chewing ☐	______	Stomach Pain ☐	______	Vaginal Discharge ☐	______
Neck Pain/Swelling ☐	______	Constipation ☐	______	Joint/Leg/Arm Pain ☐	______
Runny Nose ☐	______	Vomiting ☐	______	Easy Bruising ☐	______
Eye Drainage/Redness ☐	______	Diarrhea ☐	______	Yellow Skin/Jaundice ☐	______
Trouble Hearing ☐	______	Blood in Stool ☐	______	Rash/Skin Problems ☐	______

☐ Other ________

* Please continue on back if you are a new patient or a returning patient with changes to any section on the back.

Hospital name	

Patient Information ⑥ 한글본

초진 환자나 예전과 다르게 변한 사항이 있으신 분은 다음 장을 기록하십시오

어린이 병력

자녀가 조산이었나요, 만산이었나요? □만산 □조산 조산인 경우 몇 주 일찍? ____________

임신중 혹은 출산 시 문제가 있었나요? □아니오 □네 만약 '네'라면 설명하십시오 ____________

출생시 몸무게는?____________출산 후 병원에 며칠간 있었나요?____________

자녀가 병원에 입원한 일이 있었나요? □아니오 □네 만약 '네'라면 설명하십시오 ____________

자녀가 수술을 받은 일이 있었나요? □아니오 □네 만약 '네'라면 설명하십시오 ____________

자녀가 갖고 있는 만성적 증세가 있었나요? □아니오 □네 만약 '네'라면 설명하십시오 ____________

자녀에게 알레르기가 있나요(약/음식/그 외)? □아니오 □네 만약 '네'라면 설명하십시오 ____________

자녀의 예방접종을 담당하는 주치의가 있나요? □아니오 □네 ____________

발육/학교

자녀에게 육체적 정신적 성장 심리상태 혹은 발달의 문제가 있나요? □아니오 □네 만약 '네'라면 설명하십시오 ____________

자녀가 학교나 공부에 어려움이 있나요? □아니오 □네 만약 '네'라면 설명하십시오 ____________

가족 병력

가족 구성원이 갖고 있는 증세에 표시하세요.

증세	가족 구성원	증세	가족 구성원
심장질환/고혈압/뇌졸중	________	간질 혹은 두통	________
폐질환/천식	________	소아관절염	________
출혈 문제/암/종양	________	그 외 다른 병력,	
신장질환 혹은 당뇨병	________	질환, 조기사망	________
위 혹은 장 질환	________		

다음 페이지 넘겨 완성하시오

Page 1

PLEASE COMPLETE IF YOU ARE A NEW PATIENT OR RETURNING PATIENT WITH CHANGES

CHILD'S HEALTH HISTORY

Was your child born early or on time?	☐On time ☐Early If early, how many weeks early? ____________
Were there any problems in the pregnancy or delivery?	☐No ☐Yes If yes, please describe below: ____________

How much did your child weight at birth?____________ How many days did your child stay in the hospital after birth?____________

Has your child ever been hospitalized?	☐No ☐Yes If yes, please describe below: ____________
Has your child had any operations?	☐No ☐Yes If yes, please describe below: ____________
Does your child have any other chronic conditions?	☐No ☐Yes If yes, please describe below: ____________
Is your child allergic to anything(medicines, food, other)?	☐No ☐Yes If yes, please describe below: ____________
Do you have a primary care provider that handles your child's immunizations?	☐No ☐Yes ____________

DEVELOPMENT/SCHOOL

Are there any concerns with your child's physical or mental development, mood, or behavior?	☐No ☐Yes If yes, please describe below: ____________
Is your child having a hard time with school or studying?	☐No ☐Yes If yes, please describe below: ____________

FAMILY HISTORY

Circle the condition and identify family members who have any of the following:

Condition	*Family member*	*Condition*	*Family member*
Heart Disease/High Blood Pressure/Stroke:	____________	Seizures or Headaches:	____________
Lung Disease/Asthma:	____________	Arthritis at a young age:	____________
Bleeding Problems/Cancer/Tumors:	____________	Any other history of family illnesses, diseases, early deaths?	____________
Kidney Disease or Diabetes:	____________		
Stomach or Intestine Disease:	____________		

PLEASE TURN OVER TO COMPLETE

Page 1

Patient Information ⑦ 한글본

가정환경

가정에 아픈 사람이 있나요? □아니오 □네
있다면 무슨 병입니까? 설명하세요
____

집에 애완동물이나 다른 동물들이 있습니까? □아니오 □네 종류기입:__________

식구 중 최근 외국을 여행한 사람이 있습니까? □아니오 □네 '네'이면 아래 기입하세요
어디?__________ 언제?__________

자녀의 출생국은 어느 나라입니까 ? □아니오 □네 '네'이면 아래 기입하세요
누구?__________ 어느 나라?__________

가정에 결핵이나 그 외 다른 감염자가 있습니까? □아니오 □네 '네'이면 기입하세요
누구?__________

가정에 흡연자가 있습니까? □아니오 □네

집에 나무를 때는 난로가 있습니까? □아니오 □네

어떤 종류의 물을 사용합니까? □수도물 □우물물

자녀의 의료정보를 어떤 방법으로 받기를 원하십니까?

□읽기(문서 혹은 도표) □듣기(개인 상담)
□보기(실물 설명) □체험(실습)

당신 외에 누가 자녀를 돌봅니까?__________

저희가 당신의 자녀와 가족을 더 효과적으로 돌보는 데 관계가 되는 다른 요구(육체적 기능, 문화적·종교적 필요사항)가 있으십니까?__________

의사 서명__________

Page 2

Patient Information ⑦ 영문본

HOME ENVIRONMENT

Is anyone living in the home sick?	☐No ☐Yes If yes, what are they sick with? Please describe below ______________________________
Are there pets or animals in the home?	☐No ☐Yes List types:____________
Has anyone in the home traveled outside the country recently?	☐No ☐Yes If yes please list below Where?________ When?________
Where you or your child born in a country?	☐No ☐Yes If yes please list below Who?________ What country?________
Does anyone in the home have TB(tuberculosis)or other infection?	☐No ☐Yes If yes who?________________
Does anyone smoke at home?	☐No ☐Yes
Is here a wood stove in the home?	☐No ☐Yes
What type of water do you have?	☐City water ☐Well water

PATIENT EDUCATION

In What ways do you prefer to learn about how to care for your child's medical needs?

☐Reading(written materials or pictures) ☐Listening(one-on-one conversation)

☐Watching(demonstration) ☐Doing(practicing myself)

Who else helps care for your child?______________________________

Do you have any needs(physical abilities, cultural, religion) related to your child's care that will help us work together better with your child and family? If so, please explain:____________________

Physicians Signature ______________________________

Page 2

Patient Questionnaire 내과 ① 한글본

내과

내과 문진표

해당 항목에 ✔를 해주세요　　　　　　　　　　　　　년　　　　월　　　　일

이름　　　　　　　　　　□남　□여
생년월일 ________ 년 ________ 월 ________ 일

주소　　　　　　　　　　전화번호

의료보험증을 가지고 있습니까?
□아니오　　　　□네

국적

어디에 어떤 이상이 있었습니까?

□열이 있다(　　　　　℃)　　　　□목이 아프다
□두통　　□가슴이 아프다　　□복통
□위통　　□두근거림　　□숨이 차다
□기침　　□목이 마르다　　□현기증
□부종　　□저린다　　□발진
□가슴에(생략) 압박감　　□구역질, 메스껍다　　□복부팽만감
□구토　　□설사　　□혈변
□식욕부진　　□고혈압　　□쉽게 피곤해진다
□체중감소　　□나른하다　　□그 외

* 언제부터 입니까?
________ 년 ________ 월 ________ 일

약이나 음식물로 알레르기를 일으킨 적이 있습니까?
□아니오　　□네 → □약　　□음식물　　□그 외

현재 복용 중인 약이 있습니까?
□아니오　　□네 → 지금 가지고 있다면 보여 주세요

현재 임신중입니까? 임신일 가능성이 있습니까?
□아니오　　□네 → ______ 개월

최종 월경
______ 년 ______ 월 ______ 일

지금까지 어떤 병을 앓았습니까?

□위장질환　　□간장질환　　□신장질환　　□심장질환
□폐의 질환　　□당뇨병　　□고혈압증　　□결핵
□천식　　□매독　　□에이즈　　□그 외

* 그 병은 다 나았습니까?　　□아니오　　□네

수혈을 받은 적이 있습니까?
□아니오　　□네

지금까지 수술을 받은 적이 있습니까?
□아니오　　□네 → 연령 ______ 세 ________ 개월

* http://www.k-i-a.or.jp/medical/

Patient Questionnaire 내과 ① 영문본

Internal Medicine

Internal Medicine Patient's Questionnaire

Please ✔mark on the appropriate heading 년 월 일

Name ☐M ☐F
DOB ________Y ________M ________D

Address Phone

Do you have health insurance?
☐No ☐Yes

Nationality

What kind of symptoms do you have?

☐fever(℃)		☐sore throat
☐headache	☐heart aches	☐abdominal pain
☐stomach pain	☐palpitation	☐short of breath
☐cough	☐thirst	☐dizziness
☐swelling	☐muscle cramps	☐rash
☐chest tightness	☐nausea	☐bloating
☐vomit	☐diarrhea	☐blood in stool
☐poor appetite	☐hypertension	☐fatigue
☐loss of weight	☐drowsy	☐other

* When did symptom start?
________Y ________M ________D

Are you allergic to any medication of food?
☐No ☐Yes → ☐medication ☐food ☐other

Are you currently taking any medicine?
☐No ☐Yes → If you now have any medicine with you, please show us

Are you pregnant? Do you think you might be pregnant?
☐No ☐Yes → ________Month

When was your last period?
________Y ________M ________D

What kind of symptoms did you have in the past?

☐stomach disease	☐intestine disease	☐renal disease	☐heart disease
☐lung disease	☐diabetes	☐hypertension	☐tuberculosis
☐asthma	☐syphilis	☐AIDS	☐other

* Are you cured of that disease? ☐No ☐Yes

Have you had blood transfusion?
☐No ☐Yes

Have you had surgery?
☐No ☐Yes → Age________Year ________Months

* http://www.k-i-a.or.jp/medical/

Patient Questionnaire 외과 ② 한글본

외과

외과 문진표

해당 항목에 ✔를 해주세요 년 월 일

이름 □남 □여
생년월일__________년 __________월 __________일

주소 전화번호

의료보험증을 가지고 있습니까?
□아니오 □네

국적

어디에 어떤 이상이 있었습니까?

□배 □위 □장 □탈장(헤르니아)
□폐 □담석 □치질 □덩어리
□배꼽 □혈변 □상처 □피부 □체중 감소
□목 □목(갑상선) □유방 □그 외

* 아픈 곳에 ○을 표해 주세요

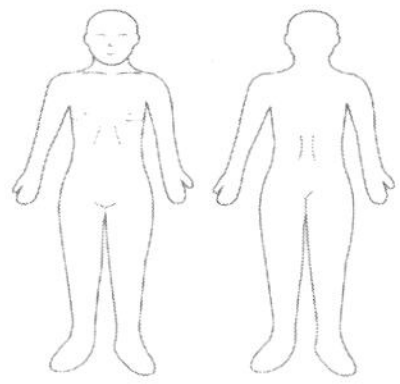

* 언제부터입니까?
______________년 ________________월 ___________________일

복통이라고 답하신 분만 써 주십시오
* 어디가 아픕니까?
□상복부 □오른쪽 하복부 □왼쪽 하복부 □하복부 전체
* 마지막으로 식사를 한 시간은 _____월_______일________시

약이나 음식물로 알레르기를 일으킨 적이 있습니까? □아니오 □네 → □약 □음식물 □그 외

현재 복용 중인 약이 있습니까? □아니오 □네 → 지금 가지고 있다면 보여 주세요

현재 임신중입니까? 임신일 가능성이 있습니까? □아니오 □네 → ________개월

지금까지 어떤 병을 앓았습니까?
□간장병 □신장병 □심장병 □결핵
□당뇨병 □천식 □고혈압 □갑상선
□에이즈 □그 외
* 그 병은 다 나았습니까? □아니오 □네

수혈을 받은 적이 있습니까?
□아니오 □네

지금까지 수술을 받은 적이 있습니까?
□아니오 □네 → 연령________세 _____________개월

소개장이 있는 분만 써 주십시오
* 차용 렌트겐필름을 가지고 계십니까?
□아니오 □네
* 차용 내시경필름을 가지고 계십니까?
□아니오 □네

* http://www.k-i-a.or.jp/medical/

Patient Questionnaire 외과 ② 영문본

Surgery

Surgery Patient's Questionnaire

Please ✔mark on the appropriate heading 년 월 일

Name ☐M ☐F
DOB __________Y __________M __________D

Address Phone

Do you have health insurance?
☐No ☐Yes

Nationality

What kind of symptoms do you have?

☐abdomen ☐stomach ☐colon/intestine ☐hernia
☐lung ☐gall stone ☐hemorrhoids ☐mass
☐navel ☐blood stool ☐skin ☐weight loss
☐neck ☐scar ☐thyroid ☐breast ☐other

* Please mark o where you feel pain

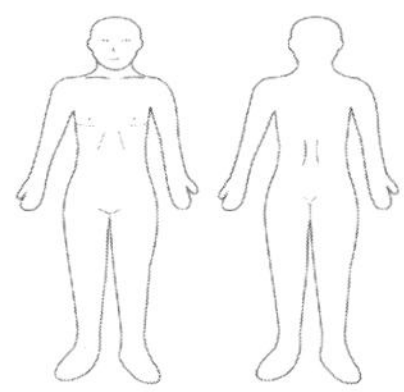

* When did the symptom start??
______________Y ________________M ____________________D

If you have abdominal pain, please fill out questions below
* Where is the pain?
☐upper abdomen ☐right lover abdominal ☐left lower abdomen
☐lower abdomen
* time of last meal ______Month_______Date_________Time

Have you ever had allergic reaction to any food or medicine?
☐No ☐Yes → ☐Medicine ☐Food ☐other

Are you taking any medicine? ☐No ☐Yes → If you have it, please show me

Are you pregnant? Is there any possibility of being pregnant? ☐No ☐Yes → _________month

Have you ever had any disease in the past?
☐liver disease ☐kidney disease ☐heart disease ☐tuberculosis
☐diabetes ☐asthma ☐hypertension ☐thyroid
☐AIDS ☐other
* Are you fully recovered from the disease?

Have you ever been transfused before?
☐No ☐Yes

Have you ever had the surgery?
☐No ☐Yes → Age_________Year ______________Month

Please fill out when you have referral
* Do you have X-ray? ☐No ☐Yes
* Do you have film with you? ☐No ☐Yes

* http://www.k-i-a.or.jp/medical/

Patient Questionnaire 피부과 ③ 한글본

피부과

피부과 문진표

해당 항목에 ✔를 해주세요　　　　　　　　　　　　　　　　　　　　년　　　　월　　　　일

이름　　　　　　　　　　　　　　　　　　□남　□여
　　　　　　　　　　　　　　　　　　　　생년월일 ________ 년 ________ 월 ________ 일

주소　　　　　　　　　　　　　　　　　　전화번호

의료보험증을 가지고 있습니까?
　　　　□아니오　　　　　　　　□네

국적

어디에 어떤 이상이 있었습니까?

□아프다　　　　　　□무좀　　　　　　* 아픈 곳에 ○을 표해 주세요
□가려움　　　　　　□화상
□발진　　　　　　　□습진
□점　　　　　　　　□멍
□상처　　　　　　　□그 외
□곪아서 짓무름
□기미

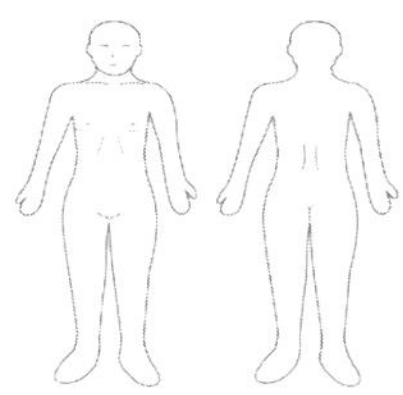

* 언제부터입니까?　　　　____년 ____월 ____일
* 증상이 변하고 있습니까?　　□아니오　　　□네

약이나 음식물로 알레르기를 일으킨 적이 있습니까?
　　　□아니오　　□네 → □약　□음식물　　　□그 외

현재 복용 중인 약이 있습니까?
　　　□아니오　　　　□네 → 지금 가지고 있다면 보여 주세요

현재 임신중입니까? 임신일 가능성이 있습니까?　□아니오　　　□네 → ______개월

최종월경　　　　____년 ____월 ____일

지금까지 어떤 병을 앓았습니까?

□위장질환	□간장질환	□신장질환	□심장질환
□폐의 질환	□당뇨병	□고혈압증	□결핵
□천식	□매독	□에이즈	□그 외

* 그 병은 다 나았습니까?　　□아니오　　　　　　□네

지금까지 수술을 받은 적이 있습니까?
　　　□아니오　　　　□네 → 연령______세 __________개월

* http://www.k-i-a.or.jp/medical/

Patient Questionnaire 피부과 ③ 영문본

Dermatology

Dermatology Patient Questionnaire

Please ✔mark on the appropriate heading 년 월 일

Name ☐M ☐F
DOB ______Y ______M ______D

Address Phone

Do you have health insurance?
☐No ☐Yes

Nationality

What kind of symptoms do you have?

☐pain ☐Athlete's food
☐itch ☐burn
☐rash ☐eczema
☐mole ☐bruise
☐scar ☐other
☐fester
☐freckles

* When did the symptom start? ______Y ______M ______D
* Do you change your symptom? ☐No ☐Yes

* Please mark o where you feel pain

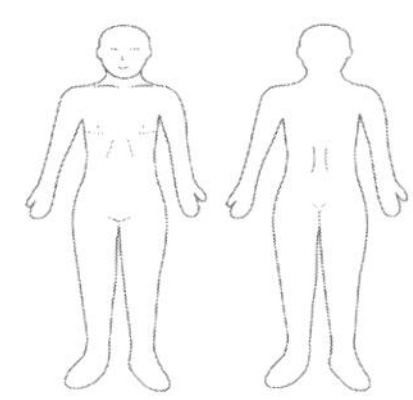

Are you allergic to any medication of food?
☐No ☐Yes → ☐medication ☐food ☐other

Are you currently taking any medicine?
☐No ☐Yes → If you now have any medicine with you, please show us

Are you pregnant? Do you think you might be pregnant? ☐No ☐Yes → ________Month

When was your last period? ______Y ______M ______D

What kind of symptoms did you have in the past?

☐stomach disease ☐intestine disease ☐renal disease ☐heart disease
☐lung disease ☐diabetes ☐hypertension ☐tuberculosis
☐asthma ☐syphilis ☐AIDS ☐other

* Are you cured of that disease? ☐No ☐Yes

Have you had ssurgery?
☐No ☐Yes → Age________Year ____________Months

* http://www.k-i-a.or.jp/medical/

산부인과

산부인과 문진표

해당 항목에 ✔를 해주세요 　　　　　　　　　년　　　월　　　일

이름　　　　　　　　　생년월일__________년 __________월 __________일

주소　　　　　　　　　전화번호

의료보험증을 가지고 있습니까?　□아니오　□네

국적

어디에 어떤 이상이 있었습니까?
□임신　□생리불순　□대하　□복통
□빈혈　□종양　□난소종양
□자궁근종　□성기출혈　□성기의 가려움증
□불임증　□자궁암 검사　□그 외

월경에 대해서
* 첫 생리는 언제였습니까? 연령 ______세　* 폐경은 언제였습니까? 연령 _________세
* 생리는 순조롭습니까? □아니오 □네　* 생리주기 □28일형 □30일형 □___일형 □불순
* 생리지속기간 ________ _____일간　* 생리양 □많다 □보통 □적다
* 생리통 □아니오 □네 → □하복부 □요통 □그 외
* 최종 월경은 언제부터 ____________년______________월________________일________________일간

임신경력 □임신 _________회
□분만 _________회 → □정상분만 ____________회 □이상분만 ____________회
□유산 _________회 → □자연유산 ____________회 □인공유산 ____________회
□그 외 ___________ → □자궁외 임신 _________회 □포상기태 ____________회

임산부는 당 병원에서 낳을 것을 희망합니까? □아니오　□네

약이나 음식물로 알레르기를 일으킨 적이 있습니까? □아니오 □네 → □약 □음식물 □그 외

현재 복용 중인 약이 있습니까? □아니오 □네 → 지금 가지고 있다면 보여 주세요

과거에 암 검사를 받은 적이 있습니까? □아니오 □네 → ________년_______월_______일

지금까지 걸린병
□간장병　□류머티스　□에이즈　□심장병　□결핵
□성병　□신장병　□그 외　□고혈압　□충수염
* 그 병은 다 나았습니까? □아니오　□네

지금까지 수술을 받은 적이 있습니까? □아니오 □네 → 연령________세_________개월

수혈을 받은 적이 있습니까?　□아니오 □네

가족에 관해

	연령	건강	건강하지 않음	유전병	고혈압	당뇨병	암
친아버지		□	□	□	□	□	□
친어머니		□	□	□	□	□	□
형제		□	□	□	□	□	□
자매		□	□	□	□	□	□
남편		□	□	□	□	□	□
자식		□	□	□	□	□	□

* http://www.k-i-a.or.jp/medical/

Patient Questionnaire 산부인과 ④ 영문본

Ob-Gyn

Ob–Gyn Patient Questionnaire

Please ✔mark on the appropriate heading 년 월 일

Name	DOB ________Y ____________M ________D
Address	Phone
Do you have health insurance?	☐No ☐Yes
Nationality	

What kind of symptoms do you have?
☐become pregnant ☐irregular period ☐vaginal discharge ☐abdominal pain
☐anemia ☐tumor ☐ovarian tumor
☐fibroids ☐genital bleeding ☐genital itch
☐infertility ☐pepsmear ☐other

About period
* When was your first period? age _____years * When was your menopause? age _____years
* Is your period smooth? ☐No ☐Yes * menstrual cycle ☐28days ☐30days ☐_____days ☐irregular
* menstrual periods ________ _____days * amount of blood loss per period ☐heavy ☐normal ☐light
* menstrual cramps ☐No ☐Yes → ☐lower abdomen ☐back pain ☐other
* When was your last peoriod? from when______year_______month______day for_______ days

Pregnancy History ☐pregnancy _________times
☐delivery _______times → ☐normal _________times ☐abnormal __________times
☐carriage _______times → ☐miscarriage _______times ☐abortion __________times
☐other _______ → ☐ectopic pregnancy _______times ☐hydatidiform Mole __________times

Are you planning to deliver at this hospital? ☐No ☐Yes

Have you every had allergic reaction to any medicine or food?
☐No ☐Yes → ☐Medicine ☐Food ☐Other

Are you currently taking any medicine? ☐No ☐Yes → Please show me if you have it with you now

Have you ever had cancer test before? ☐No ☐Yes→_______Y_______M_______D

Disease you had before
☐Liver Disease ☐Rheumatism ☐AIDS ☐Heart Disease ☐Tuberculosis
☐STD(Sexually Transmitted Disease) ☐Kidney Disease ☐Other ☐Hypertension ☐Appendicitis
* Are you fully recovered from the disease? ☐No ☐Yes

Have you ever had the surgery before? ☐No ☐Yes → Age_______Years________Months

Have you ever be transfused before? ☐No ☐Yes

Family History

	Age	Healthy	Not Healthy	Genetic Disease	Hypertension	Diabetes	Cancer
Genetic Father		☐	☐	☐	☐	☐	☐
Genetic Mother		☐	☐	☐	☐	☐	☐
Brother		☐	☐	☐	☐	☐	☐
Sister		☐	☐	☐	☐	☐	☐
Husband		☐	☐	☐	☐	☐	☐
Children		☐	☐	☐	☐	☐	☐

* http://www.k-i-a.or.jp/medical/

Patient Questionnaire 치과 ⑤ 한글본

치과

치과 문진표

해당 항목에 ✔를 해주세요 년 월 일

이름	□남 □여 생년월일_______년 _______월 _______일
주소	전화번호
의료보험증을 가지고 있습니까?	□아니오 □네
국적	

어디에 어떤 이상이 있었습니까?
□이가 아프다 □잇몸 문제 □입냄새
□충치 치료 □이를 때웠던 것이 빠짐
□치열 교정 □치석제거
□의치가 망가짐 □의치(틀니)를 만들고 싶음
□검진 □그 외

약이나 음식물로 알레르기를 일으킨 적이 있습니까?
□아니오 □네 → □약 □음식물 □그 외

현재 복용 중인 약이 있습니까?
□아니오 □네 → 지금 가지고 있다면 보여 주세요

마취를 한 적이 있습니까? □아니오 □네

이를 뽑은 적이 있습니까? □아니오 □네

현재 임신중입니까? 임신일 가능성이 있습니까?
□아니오 □네 → ______개월

과거에 암 검사를 받은 적이 있습니까?
□아니오 □네 → _______년 ______월 ______일

지금까지 어떤 병을 앓았습니까?
□위장질환 □간장질환 □신장질환 □심장질환
□폐의 질환 □당뇨병 □고혈압증 □결핵
□천식 □매독 □에이즈 □그 외
*그 병은 다 나았습니까? □아니오 □네

어떤 치료를 원하십니까?
□나쁜 부분은 전부 치료하고 싶다
□지금 아픈 이빨만 치료하고 싶다
□보험범위 내에서 치료하고 싶다
□사비진료라도 상관없다
□상담해서 결정하고 싶다

* http://www.k-i-a.or.jp/medical/

Patient Questionnaire 치과 ⑤ 영문본

Dentistry

Dentistry Patient Questionnaire

Please ✔mark on the appropriate heading 년 월 일

Name ☐M ☐F
DOB__________Y ______________M __________D

Address Phone

Do you have health insurance? ☐No ☐Yes

Nationality

What kind of symptoms do you have?

☐tooth pain ☐gum problem ☐breath smell
☐cavity treatment ☐loose crown
☐orthodontic consultation ☐scaling
☐broken denture ☐need new denture
☐regular check-up ☐other

Have you every had allergic reaction to any medicine or food?
☐No ☐Yes → ☐Medicine ☐Food ☐Other

Are you currently taking any medicine?
☐No ☐Yes → Please show me if you have it with you now

Have you ever be under anesthesia? ☐No ☐Yes

Have your teeth been extracted? ☐No ☐Yes

Are you currently pregnant? Are you eligible for being pregnant?
☐No ☐Yes → ______Months

Have you had cancer test before?
☐No ☐Yes → _______Y______M______D

What kind of symptoms did you have in the past?

☐abdominal disease ☐liver disease ☐kidney disease ☐heart disease
☐lung disease ☐diabetes ☐Hypertension ☐tuberculosis
☐asthma ☐syphilis ☐AIDS ☐other

* Are you cured of that disease? ☐No ☐Yes

What kind of treatment would you like to receive?

☐I want to receive treatments for all the problems
☐I want a treatment for my painful tooth
☐I want to receive the treatment only which is covered by my insurance
☐I do not mind paying my own
☐I want to decide after the consultation

* http://www.k-i-a.or.jp/medical/

Patient Questionnaire 안과 ⑥ 한글본

안과

안과 문진표

해당 항목에 ✔를 해주세요　　　　　　　　　　　　　년　　　　월　　　　일

이름	□남 □여 생년월일__________년 __________월 __________일
주소	전화번호
의료보험증을 가지고 있습니까?	□아니오　　　　□네
국적	

어디에 어떤 이상이 있었습니까?

□오른쪽 눈　□왼쪽 눈　□양쪽 다
□눈곱이 낀다　□눈물이 나온다　□눈이 아프다
□다래끼　□희미하게 보인다　□눈부시다
□꺼끌꺼끌하다　□물건이 이중으로 보인다
□그 외

* 언제부터입니까? __________년 __________월 __________일

약이나 음식물로 알레르기를 일으킨 적이 있습니까?
□아니오　□네 → □약　□음식물　□그 외

현재 복용 중인 약이 있습니까?
□아니오　□네 → 지금 가지고 있다면 보여 주세요

마취를 한 적이 있습니까?
□아니오　□네

지금까지 어떤 병을 앓았습니까?

□복부질환　□간장병　□심장병
□폐의 질환　□에이즈　□당뇨병
□고혈압증　□매독　□그 외

* 그 병은 다 나았습니까?　□아니오　□네

가족 중에 눈병인 사람이 있습니까?
□없다　□있다 → 누가?__________
어떤?__________

* http://www.k-i-a.or.jp/medical/

Patient Questionnaire 안과 ⑥ 영문본

Opthalmology

Opthalmology Patient Questionnaire

Please ✔mark on the appropriate heading 년 월 일

Name ☐M ☐F
DOB__________Y ______________M __________D

Address Phone

Do you have health insurance? ☐No ☐Yes

Nationality

What kind of symptoms do you have?

☐right eye	☐left eye	☐both eyes
☐eye mucus	☐tears/watery eye	☐pain in the eye
☐sty	☐blurry vision	☐sensitive to light
☐(irritably)rough	☐double vision	
☐others		

* When did this problem start? ______________ Y ______________ M __________________ D

Have you every had allergic reaction to any medicine or food?
☐No ☐Yes → ☐Medicine ☐Food ☐Other

Are you currently taking any medicine?
☐No ☐Yes → Please show me if you have it with you now

Have you ever be under anesthesia?
☐No ☐Yes

What kind of symptoms did you have in the past?

☐abdominal disease	☐liver disease	☐heart disease
☐lung disease	☐AIDS	☐diabetes
☐hypertension	☐syphilis	☐other

* Are you cured of that disease? ☐No ☐Yes

Does any of your family member have eye disease?
☐No ☐Yes → Who?________________________
What kind?________________________

* http://www.k-i-a.or.jp/medical/

3. 환자 진료기록과 그 외(Medical Chart Notes, etc.)

외국인이 국내에서 의료서비스를 받게 되면 치료를 받는 동안 모든 내용을 문서화하여야 하며 출국과 함께 모든 환자와 관련된 서류들을 본인이 가져갈 수 있도록 해주어야 한다. 특히 환자의 진료 내용은 가장 중요한 서류이며 환자의 자국어로 정확하게 번역된 합법적 자료이어야만 한다.

■ 정의(Definition)

환자 차트라고도 불리는 환자의 진찰기록은 문서(paper documents)로 혹은 전자 문서(electronic documents)로 기록·보관된다. 전자 문서에는 전자 진료기록(electronic medical records)과 오디오나 비디오기록(audio video tapes), 영상(images) 등이 포함된다. 환자의 자세하고 광범위한 진료 내용이 포함된다.

■ 목적(Purpose)

환자의 건강 상태, 진단과 치료, 검사 및 치료에 따른 변화 등을 기록하여 환자를 여러 가지 측면에서 관찰하고 일관성 있고 보다 나은 치료를 제공할 수 있도록 한다.

■ 내용(Description)

환자 차트는 환자와 관계되는 모든 의료정보를 포함한다. 의료기관마다 조금씩 다른 형식을 사용하기도 하지만 차트의 목적을 달성하기 위한 공통적인 내용을 갖게 된다.

컴퓨터 기술의 발전과 광범위한 보급에 따라 보다 많은 곳에서 전자 정보 시스템을 사용하며 이에 따라 정보 접근의 정확성과 편리성, 그리고 기록보관의 효율성이 증대되었다. 이 정보는 환자 자신의 개인적 정보이므로 문서 형태의 차트이든 전자 정보 시스템이든 의료기관은 기밀을 유지할 수 있어야만 한다.

차트는 대부분의 경우 의사나 간호사가 기록한다. 의사는 진찰 내용(examination)과 진단(diagnosis), 예후(prognosis), 치료방법의 결정과 내용 등을 기록하고 간호사는 환자의 상태와 치료에 따른 변화, 병의 진행 등을 기록한다.

그 외에 의사의 요청이나 허락에 따라 사회복지사, 심리상담가, 영양사, 물리치료사 등의 의료진이 환자 차트를 볼 수 있게 된다.

또한 법적인 이유나 혹은 보험 관계와 관련되어 공개될 때도 있다.

그러나 이러한 예외적인 경우를 제외하고는, 환자 차트는 철저히 기밀성이 지켜지고 노출이 제한되도록 규정되어 있어야 한다.

따라서 문서화된 차트는 일정 장소에 안전하게 보관되어야 하며, 전자 시스템의 경우에도 여러 가지 보안 시스템을 구축하여 노출이 제한되어야 한다. 정부나 병원의 규정에 따라 마약 사용자, 정신 질환자, 에이즈와 같은 전염병 환자의 경우 그 사실을 기관에 알게 한다. 그러나 이 정보는 불필요한 노출이 없도록 철저히 통제되고 보관된다.

환자에게는 이 모든 정보에 언제든지 접근할 수 있도록 해주어야 하며, 만약 응급 시 또는 어떠한 이유로든 이 정보가 필요한 경우 환자나 환자의 법적 보호자의 동의서(written permission to release records)가 있어야 한다.

환자의 진료기록인 차트는 일관성 있는 치료에 반드시 필요한 자료이다. 외국인 환자가 국내에서 치료를 받게 되면 치료 내용을 바탕으로 본국에서 계속적인 치료를 받을 수 있도록 번역된 차트를 제공해 주어야 한다.

1) 환자 의료기록(Patient Chart Note) 작성

차트는 환자의 치료가 이루어지는 순간부터 기록된다. 치료가 한 장소에서만 이루어지는 것이 아니므로 이 기록은 일관성을 유지할 수 있도록 환자가 방문하는 모든 시설에서 환자의 동의(request permission to obtain copies of previous records) 하에 공유하게 된다. 차트에는 다음과 같은 것이 포함된다.

(1) 초진 때 작성하는 기록(Initial Chart Note)의 내용

• 주요 증상(Chief Complaint): 환자가 치료받고자 하는 증상이 무엇인지, 즉 병원을 찾은 주요 이유를 말한다.

□ I woke up this morning with some chest pain, shortness of breath and felt a little dizzy.

오늘 아침 일어났을 때 가슴 통증과 숨가쁨, 그리고 조금 어지러움을 느꼈습니다.

☐ I have had stomach pain, diarrhea, vomiting and fever for two days.

지난 이틀 동안 복통, 설사, 구토 증상과 열이 있었습니다.

☐ I had lacerations, left hand.

왼쪽 손에 열상(찢어진 상처)을 입었습니다.

• 병의 내력(History of Present Illness): 환자의 증상과 관련하여 여러 가지 질의응답 내용, 진찰 내용(문진, 촉진) 등을 포함한다.

☐ This 37 year old female experience similar symptoms last month but was not as serious as she feel this morning. She is diabetic.

이 37세의 여성 환자는 지난달 비슷한 증세를 경험하였으나 오늘만큼 심하지는 않았습니다. 이 환자는 당뇨병이 있습니다.

☐ This 26 year-old male who cut his left middle finger on a pocket knife while attempting to cut a piece of duct tape. He is generally in good health.

이 26세의 남성 환자는 도관용 테이프를 포켓용 칼로 자르다가 왼쪽 중지를 베었습니다. 일반적으로 건강은 양호합니다.

• 진료 및 수술 경력(Past Medical & Surgical History):

- 치료기록(Treatment Record: 환자가 받은 모든 치료 내력)
- 수술받은 기록(Surgical History)
- 진료기록(Procedures: 병의 증상에 대한 여러 가지 의학적인 처치 및 절차)
- 장 내시경 혹은 심장 절개 수술 등 모든 진료기록(Therapeutic and Diagnostic Procedures)
- 약 복용기록(Medication Record: 환자의 모든 약복용 내력)
- 가족의 건강 상태(유전적 요소)
- 현재 종사하는 일, 사회적 환경(Social)
- 흡연, 알코올 습관, 알레르기 등에 대해서도 기록한다.

☐ Hip replacement surgery in 1998

1998년 고관절 치환 수술

☐ She has chronic back pain.

그녀는 만성적 요통이 있다.

☐ Patient's father died at age 75. He had diabetes and a heart condition.

환자의 아버지는 75세에 돌아가셨다. 그는 당뇨병과 심장 문제를 가지고 있었다.

☐ Patient is taking ibuprofen last 2 days.

환자는 지난 2일간 이부프로펜(만성관절 류머티즘 따위의 치료에 쓰이는 비스테로이드성 소염진통제)을 복용하고 있다.

☐ Patient is allergic to Penicillin.

환자는 페니실린에 알레르기 반응을 갖고 있다.

☐ Patient is smoking 1 pack a day.

환자는 하루에 한 갑씩 담배를 핀다.

• 기관별 검토(Review of the System)

☐ HEENT: Head, Eyes, Ears, Nose, Throat	☐ 머리, 눈, 귀, 코, 목(두부 및 이비인후 계통)
☐ Respiratory	☐ 호흡기 계통
☐ Cardiovascular	☐ 심장계통
☐ Gastrointestinal	☐ 소화기 계통
☐ Genitourinary	☐ 비뇨생식기 계통
☐ Neurologic	☐ 신경계통
☐ Psychiatric	☐ 정신계통
☐ Musculoskeletal	☐ 골근육계통

☐ HEENT within normal limits

머리, 눈, 귀, 코, 목 정상(범위 안에 속한다)

☐ Thorax and lungs no rales or rhonchi

가슴과 폐 수포음 없음

☐ Cardiovascular no murmurs

심장 잡음 없음

☐ Physical Examination	☐ 신체검사
☐ General Appearance	☐ 일반 외형
☐ 생명의 징후(Vital Signs)	☐ 맥박(Pulse), 호흡수(Respiratory Rate), 혈압(Blood Pressure), 체온(Body Temp)

☐ Skin	☐ 피부
☐ 가슴(Chest)	☐ 심장박동(Heart), 폐(Lungs), 유방(Breast-Optional)
☐ Abdomen	☐ 배
☐ Extremities/Motion	☐ 사지 움직임
☐ Pelvic-Optional	☐ 골반
☐ Diagnostic Studies and Diagnosis	☐ 진단

- 치료를 위한 지시사항(Orders): 약복용에 대한 의사의 지시사항과 여러 가지 치료 및 검사 주문 등에 대한 내용
- 상담기록(Consultations): 환자, 환자 가족과 의료진 간의 모든 상담내용 기록
- 향후(Care Plans): 치료의 목표 설정과 그에 따른 계획(의료시설 내에서의 치료 계획, 퇴원 후의 치료 계획 등)

(2) 경과기록(Progress Notes or Follow Up Notes)

경과기록(Progress Notes)은 초진 이후에 계속되는 환자 진료 과정에 대한 기록으로 의사나 간호사 등 의료진에 의해 작성된다. 병의 경과, 치료, 수술 등에 대한 내용 및 결과, 약의 복용, 입원과 퇴원 등에 대한 내용이다. 여기에는 검사기록, 수술기록, 관찰기록 등이 포함된다.

- 검사기록(Radiology and Pathology Report): 검사실에서 하는 모든 검사내용과 결과, 영상의학과에서 이루어지는 모든 검사와 그 결과 등(예: 혈액검사, 심전도 검사 등)
- 수술기록(Operative Report): 수술기록에는 다음과 같은 내용이 기록된다.

☐ Preoperative Diagnosis	☐ 수술 전 진단
☐ Postoperative Diagnosis	☐ 수술 후 진단
☐ Reason for Operation or Indications	☐ 수술 동기 혹은 의학적 증상
☐ Operation Performed or Name of Operation	☐ 수술 명
☐ Surgeon	☐ 수술 담당의

☐ Assistants	☐ 수술 보조자
☐ Anesthesiologist	☐ 마취 담당의
☐ Anesthesia	☐ 마취의 종류
☐ Indications for Procedure	☐ 처치를 위한 증상들
☐ Findings	☐ 발견 내용
☐ Procedure, Operative Course, or Technique	☐ 처치, 수술경위, 사용된 기술
☐ Complications	☐ 합병증
☐ Tourniquet Time	☐ 지혈 시간
☐ Hardware	☐ 수술에 쓰인 기구들
☐ Drains	☐ 유출 물질
☐ Specimens	☐ 피검물
☐ Estimated Blood Loss	☐ 혈액 소실양
☐ Instrument, Sponge, and Needle Counts	☐ 기구, 스폰지, 주사기 사용 수
☐ Disposition Of Patient	☐ 환자의 체질, 경향
☐ Follow Up	☐ 추적관찰

• 관찰기록(Flow Records): 계속적인 관찰이 필요한 경우 이를 지속적으로 기록해 나간다. 예를 들어, 중환자의 경우 환자의 상태, 사용되는 기구, 변화에 따른 여러 가지 조치 등을 기록하게 된다. 이런 기록은 정확하고 빠른 정보 전달과 효과적인 치료를 유도해 줄 수 있다. 데이터나 그래프를 이용하기도 한다.

(3) **퇴원기록**(Discharge Report)

환자가 병원에 입원했다가 퇴원할 때 작성한다. 다음과 같은 정보와 지시사항 등이 포함된다.

☐ Admitting Diagnosis	☐ 입원 시 진단
☐ Discharge Diagnosis	☐ 퇴원 시 진단
☐ Chief Complaint	☐ 주요 증세

☐ History or History of Present Illness	☐ 질병의 내력
☐ Hospital Course	☐ 병원 입원 내력
☐ Prognosis	☐ 병의 예후
☐ Plan, Discharge Plan, or Disposition	☐ 계획, 퇴원 계획 혹은 환자의 성향
☐ Discharge Instructions	☐ 퇴원에 따른 지시사항
☐ Condition	☐ 규정, 제한 조건

(4) 그 외

그 외에 사망 진단서(Death Summary), 혹은 서신문(Correspondence) 등이 있다.

① 차트 작성의 기본요소

환자의 차트는 환자 치료에 사용되는 여러 가지 정보를 제공하는 자료이므로 정확하고 구체적이어야만 한다. 진료가 일어나는 장소나 시간에 상관없이 이 기록이 필요하며, 모든 정보는 신뢰할 수 있는 근거와 법적 효용성을 갖고 있어야 한다. 따라서 차트 작성에는 필수적인 여러 가지 기본 요소들이 있다.

- 진료날짜와 시간을 명시한다(include date and time on all records).
- 환자 이름(full patient name), 환자 고유번호(medical record number), 생년월일(date of birth)을 기록한다.
- 내용이 여러 페이지일 경우 계속되는 것에 대해 명시하여 준다(예: continued page 2).
- 담당 의사의 사인이 있어야 한다.
- 문서의 형태인 경우 지울 수 없는 검정 펜으로 기록한다(수정이 있을 경우 수정한 기록자가 사인하여 증명한다).
- 진찰 날짜 순서대로 정리한다.
- 기록이 이유 없이 파기되지 않도록 한다.
- 약어를 쓸 경우 세계적으로 통용되는(universally accepted abbreviations) 약어만 사용하여 오해가 없도록 한다.
- 상반되는 내용이 없도록 한다(예를 들어 의사의 기록에는 환자가 복통을 호소했다고 되어 있는데 간호사가 기록할 때에 환자가 통증이 없다고 하는 경우 이 문제에 대해 확실한 사실을 밝

히고 정확히 기록하도록 한다).

- 주관적인 사실(subjective)과 객관적 사실(objective)에 대해 명백하게 구분하여 기록해야 한다.
- 환자와 관계있는 모든 사실들은 기록(documented information)이 되어야 하며 문서에 기록되지 않은 사실(undocumented information)은 법적인 효력이 없다.
- 기록이 시행된 시간과 일자를 반드시 기록한다. 만약 차후에 첨가되는 사항에 대해서는 '추가조항(addendum)' 이라고 해서 따로 기록해 두고 추가된 시간과 날짜도 기록하도록 한다.
- 환자의 말을 직접 인용할 때는 따옴표를 사용하여 구술 내용 그대로 기록한다.
- 차트는 아무데나 방치되어 권한 밖의 외부인에 의해 노출되거나 변경되는 일이 없어야 한다.
- 의료기관마다 몇 가지 다른 형식의 기록 방법을 통해 좀 더 효과적이고 정확한 길을 모색한다.

예를 들어 구술 방법에는 CBE, SOAP, PIE 등이 있다.

'CBE'란 중요한 사실, 예외적인 일들만을 기록(Charting by Exception)하여 반복을 피하고 기록하는 시간을 줄일 수 있도록 하는 방법이다. 이 경우에 관찰 기록은 따로 작성(separate flow record)하여 환자와 규칙적인 접촉을 하게 된다. 많은 의료기관에서 특별한 일이 일어나지 않아도 규칙적인 환자 의료기록이 이루어지는 것을 원칙으로 하고 있는데, 예를 들어 간호사의 근무 교대가 있을 때마다 매번 환자에 대한 관찰기록을 하도록 하고 있다.

'SOAP'는 많이 쓰이고 있는 기록 방법 중의 하나인데, 주관적 관찰 내용(Subjective), 객관적 관찰 내용(Objective), 치료 시행 내용 평가(Assessment), 치료 계획(Plan) 등의 순으로 서술한다. 즉, 환자의 신상과 의견(History), 환자의 상태에 대한 객관적인 사실들(Physical Exam), 환자 진단(Diagnosis), 그리고 미래의 치료 계획 등의 순으로 기술하는 방법이다.

- 주관적 관찰 내용(Subjective component)은 환자의 현재 상태를 서술식으로 기술한다. 또한 환자와의 상담(oral intake)을 통해 알 수 있는 환자의 건강 상태(signs and symptoms), 과거 병력(past medical history), 증세 등이 그 내용이 된다. 여러 기관의 진찰을 통해 알 수 있는 병적 증세와 과거의 건강 상태, 수술 경력, 가족의 건강 내력, 사회적 배경 등도 포함하며, 여기에 현재 복용하는 약, 과거에 복용했던 약(medications), 알레르기 반

응(allergies) 등도 기록한다.

만약 초진인 경우, 현재 증상에 대한 정보, 즉 증상의 시작(onset), 기간(duration), 상태(character), 발생 장소(location), 증세를 악화시키는 요인(alleviating/aggravating factors) 등도 첨가한다.

- 객관적 관찰 내용(Objective component)에는 생체 사인 내용(맥박수, 혈압 체온), 나이, 체중, 의사의 진찰 결과들, 검사실 결과 등이 포함된다.
- 치료 시행 내용(Assessment)은 환자의 증세에 대한 의사의 진단, 의사의 소견과 그에 따른 치료, 문제점에 대한 열거 등이다.
- 치료 계획(Plan)은 환자의 증세에 대해서 의료진이 무엇을 할 것인지에 대한 내용이다. 예를 들면, 검사 계획(labs), 방사선과적 검토(radiological work up), 약(medications)처방, 시술(procedures) 계획, 간호사 지시 사항, 환자를 다른 병원에 보내도록 계획하는 내용 등이다. 또 무엇을 논의 했고, 환자에게 어떤 지시를 했는지, 또 다음 진료를 위한 방문 계획 등에 대한 내용 등도 포함한다. 종종 치료 시행 내용과 치료 계획은 구분 없이 한꺼번에 기록하기도 한다.

SOAP 형식에 의해 작성된 차트의 예

	Surgery Service, Dr. Heigg 외과 치료, 의사 헤이그 씨
S:	No Chest Pain or Shortness of Breath. "Feeling better today." Patient reports flatus 가슴통증이나 숨가쁨 증세 없음 "오늘은 좋아졌다" 가스(방귀)를 배출했다고 환자가 말함
O:	Afebrile, P 84, R 16, BP 130/82. No acute distress. 무열, 맥박(Pulse) 84, 호흡(Respiration) 16, 혈압(Blood pressure) 130/80 급성 통증 없음
	Neck no JVD, Lungs clear 목정맥 팽만 없음, 폐 깨끗함(잡음 없음)
	Cor RRR 심장박동 정상(Coronary regular rhythm and rate)
	Abd Bowel sounds present, mild RLQ tenderness, less than yesterday. Wounds look clean 위, 장음 정상, 오른쪽 하복부에 약간의 압통, 어제보다 덜함. 상처는 깨끗함
	Ext without enema 관장 없이 배변

A:	Patient is a 37 year old man on post-operative day 2 for laparoscopic appendectomy, recently passed flatus. 환자는 37세의 남성이고 복강경 맹장 수술 후 2일째, 최근 가스(방귀)가 배출되었다.
P:	Recovering well. Advance diet. Continue to monitor labs. Prepare for discharge home tomorrow morning 잘 회복되고 있음. 규정식사를 먹게 할 것. 검사실 결과 계속 관찰. 내일 아침 퇴원 준비

그 외에 Focus charting 혹은 PIE(Problem-Intervention Evaluation) charting 방법은 어떤 특정 문제에 대하여 계속적으로 기록하는 것이다. 예를 들어 환자가 'Fluid volume deficit'라는 진단이 내려지면 이는 환자가 탈수상태라는 것을 뜻하며 이에 적합한 치료가 진행되는 동안 모든 과정을 기록하게 되는 경우이다. 탈수상태를 벗어나도록 환자가 섭취하는 음식물, 또 혈관을 통해 투여되는 주사의 종류 및 그 양, 그에 따른 변화 등을 집중적으로 기록하는 방법이다.

② 보관 및 운영(Maintenance)

대체로 의료기관의 자료실에 일정 기간 보관한다. 환자기록은 특별한 이유가 없는 한 변경될 수 없다. 환자가 자기 의료기록을 요구하면 문서 형식, 전자 정보 형식, 컴퓨터 영상, 필름 형태 등 여러 가지로 제공하게 된다.

③ 환자 진료 및 경과기록지 번역

환자의 의료 관계 서류를 번역하는 일은 여러 가지 법적(legal mecical record), 도덕적 의무(ethical responsibility)를 수반한다. 모든 내용은 변경되거나 생략되어서는 안 되며, 빠짐없이 정확하게 번역되어야 한다. 또한 모든 환자의 정보는 절대적으로 기밀성이 유지되어야만 한다. 번역한 사람이 어떠한 이유에서든 그 내용을 유출하면 법적인 책임까지 직면할 수 있음을 알고 있어야 할 것이다.

2) 의료기록의 번역

한글 차트를 영어로 번역하려면 정확한 영어 사용법을 익혀야 한다.

의료기록에 있어서도 우리가 알고 있는 문법과 같은 문법을 적용하면 된다. 이는 일상적 구문론, 언어용법 등과 그 외에 여러 가지에 법칙이 동일하게 적용된다는 것을 말한다. 의료기록은 내용의 정확성을 위해 문법에 따라 올바르게 기술되어야 하며, 전문성을 갖도록 하는 것이 중요하다. 문법적으로 올바른 표현은 올바른 단어의 사용으로 직결될 수 있으며 여기에는 여러 가지 요소가 포함된다. 바른 동사의 시제 사용은 환자의 질병이나 상태가 과거의 일인지 현재의 일인지 구별할 수 있는 근거가 된다. 이는 의사가 어떠한 치료를 할지 결정하는 데 중대한 요소이기 때문이다. 명사, 형용사, 부사 등의 사용도 환자의 진단 및 치료 결정에 절대적 영향을 준다는 것을 알고 정확성을 위해 최선을 다해야 한다.

■ 차트 번역의 일반 문법(Grammar/General Standard of Style)

이제 차트 작성 형식에 따라 문법적으로 정확하게 번역하는 데 알아두어야 할 기본 영어 사용법을 익혀 보도록 한다.

명사(Noun)

사람 이름, 장소, 사물, 생각 등

• 고유명사(Proper Noun):

☐ St. Joseph's Hospital	☐ 성요셉병원
☐ Band-Aid	☐ 밴드에이드
☐ Tylenol	☐ 타이레놀

• 보통명사(Common Noun):

☐ woman	☐ 여자
☐ Patient	☐ 환자
☐ doctor	☐ 의사

• 추상명사(Abstract Noun):

☐ strength	☐ 강도
☐ pain	☐ 통증
☐ depression	☐ 우울함

• 구상명사(Concrete Noun):

☐ chart	☐ 차트
☐ medication	☐ 약
☐ surgery	☐ 수술

• 집합명사(Collective Nouns):

☐ family	☐ 가족
☐ staff	☐ 직원
☐ couple	☐ 부부

• 복합명사(Compound Nouns):

☐ Children's Medical Center	☐ 어린이병원
☐ Fairland Cancer Treatment Clinic	☐ 페어랜드 암센터
☐ Physical Therapy Room	☐ 물리 치료실

대명사(Pronoun)

• 주격대명사(Nominative): I, you, he, she, it, we, they

☐ He had a complete blood count.

그는 혈구수 측정을 마쳤다.

☐ She is scheduled for a endoscopy.

그녀는 내시경검사 예정이다.

• 목적격대명사(Objective): me, him, her, us, them

☐ The patient need to come and see me on January of 2011.

환자는 2011년 1월 나를 보러(진찰하러) 와야 한다.

• 소유격대명사(Possessive): my, mine, your, yours, his, her, hers, its, our, ours, their, theirs

☐ The discharge instructions were given to the patient and her family.

환자와 그녀의 가족에게 퇴원 지시 내용을 알려 주었다.

☐ Her genetics indicate the potential for breast cancer.

그녀의 유전적 특징은 유방암의 가능성을 보여 준다.

• 재귀대명사(Reflexive)

☐ The patient injured himself while cutting trees in his garden.

환자는 자신의 정원에서 나무를 자르다 상처를 입었다.

☐ She insisted on dressing herself.

그녀는 스스로 옷을 입겠다고 했다.

• 강의대명사(Intensive)

☐ Victor himself was not hurt.

빅터 그 자신은 다치지 않았다.

• 관계대명사(Relative)

☐ Dr. Lim is a physician whom we can trust.

닥터임은 우리가 신뢰할 만한 의사다.

☐ The surgery was one that he had not heard of before.

그 수술에 대해 그는 전에 들어 본 적이 없다.

• 의문대명사(Interrogative)

☐ Who brought the patient to the emergency room?

누가 환자를 응급실로 데리고 왔습니까?

☐ What is the name of your primary care physician?

주치의의 성함이 무엇입니까?

• 지시대명사(Demonstrative)

☐ That is an excellent plan.

저것은 좋은 계획이다.

☐ This seems to be a minor problem.

이것은 대수롭지 않은 문제로 보인다.

• 부정대명사(Indefinite)

☐ All of us are here.
우리 모두 여기 있다.

☐ Few of the patients were new.
환자의 겨우 몇 명만 신환이다.

☐ Anyone's mistake can lead to disaster.
누군가의 실수가 큰 재난을 가져올 수 있다.

☐ No one knows how difficult her recovery has been.
아무도 그녀의 회복이 얼마나 어려운지 모른다.

☐ Each needs to be kept its own separate bottle.
각각 분리된 병에 보관되어야만 한다.

☐ Anyone that has been through this procedure needs to take a rest for a while.
이 처치(혹은 치료)를 받은 자는 누구나 잠시 휴식을 취해야 한다.

☐ Few are chosen for that position.
그런 자세를 선택하는 경우는 극히 드물다.

☐ Some of her symptoms are ambiguous.
그녀의 증세 중 일부는 명확하지 않다.

☐ Some of his pain is difficult to describe.
그의 통증 중 일부는 표현하기가 어렵다.

☐ Most of the patients follow the directions very well.
환자의 대부분은 지시를 잘 따른다.

형용사(Adjective)

어떤(What kind), (which one), (how many)

☐ foamy urine	☐ 거품이 있는 소변
☐ loose stools	☐ 설사
☐ fatty acid	☐ 지방산
☐ noncompliant patient	☐ (결정에 대해) 순응하지 않는 환자
☐ this & that treatment	☐ 이런 저런 치료

☐ numerous cells ☐ 다수의 세포

☐ several medicines ☐ 여러 가지 약

☐ two pills ☐ 두 알

☐ The patient, disoriented and confused, was unable to provide his family history.
환자는 분별하지 못하고 혼란에 빠져 있어서 그의 가족력에 대해 알려줄 수 없었다.

☐ The patient was alert and oriented.
환자는 민감하고 분별력도 있었다.

☐ Her palms and soles were red and warm.
그녀의 손바닥과 발바닥이 붉고 열이 있었다.

☐ Which medication did you give the patient?
환자에게 어떤 약을 주었습니까?

☐ I need this information.
나는 이 정보가 필요하다.

☐ Get your prescription drugs at the hospital pharmacy.
병원 약국에서 당신의 처방약을 받으세요.

☐ She had a painful bleeding ulcer.
그녀는 고통스러운 출혈성 위궤양을 앓고 있다.

동사(Verb)

• 현재형

☐ The patient has a history of mental illness.
환자는 정신 질환의 병력이 있다.

☐ The patient is to take tylenol three times a day as needed for pain.
환자는 통증이 있을 때마다 필요에 따라 하루 세 번씩 타이레놀을 먹을 것이다.

☐ He can get a prescription for the symptom.
그는 증세에 대한 처방약을 받을 수 있다.

☐ The patient reports a great deal of stress associated with caring for a parent with Alzheimer's.

환자는 치매 증세를 갖고 있는 부모를 돌보는 것과 관련하여 상당한 스트레스를 호소한다.

☐ She is in her pain.

그녀는 통증이 있다.

☐ The differential diagnosis is myocardial infarction versus costochondritis versus gastrointestinal etiology.

다른 진단은 심근 경색 대(인지) 늑연골염 대(인지) 위장의 병인(인지)이다.

☐ Her insurance requires her to have her blood work done from Center Lab.

그녀의 보험사는 그녀에게 혈액검사를 센터 검사실에서 할 것을 요청한다.

☐ The patient presents with his previous x-ray.

환자는 과거 엑스레이를 보여 준다.

☐ The patient lives at senior home with his caregiver.

환자는 그의 간병인과 함께 노인을 위한 시설에 살고 있다.

☐ The patient's wife has power of attorney for her husband's care decisions.

환자의 부인은 남편의 치료에 대한 결정에 대해 법적 권리를 갖고 있다.

☐ The patient is 5 feet 10 inches tall.

환자는 키가 5피트 10인치이다.

• 미래형

☐ He will be seen in the office on Monday.

그는 월요일 사무실에 와서 (나에게) 보일 것이다.

☐ She will return for her follow-up next month.

그녀는 다음 달 재진을 위해 다시 방문할 것이다.

☐ The patient will be referred to Northwest Cancer Center for consultation.

그 환자는 상담을 위해 노스웨스트 암센터에 보내질 것이다.

☐ He will be discharged tomorrow.

그는 내일 퇴원할 것이다.

☐ She will be given induction anesthesia prior to the procedure.

그녀는 시술 전에 유도 마취를 받게 될 것이다.

☐ He will follow up in the eye clinic two weeks later.

그는 2주 후에 안과에서 재검진을 받을 것이다.

☐ She will have her tests performed in the Hospital lab.

그녀는 병원 검사실에서 검사들을 할 것이다.

☐ The procedure will be done on July 20th this year.

시술은 올해 7월 20일 시행할 것이다.

☐ She will be transferred to the care of surgeon.

그녀는 외과의의 치료로 보내질 것이다.

☐ He will be discharged to home to rest.

그는 쉬기 위해 집으로 퇴원을 할 것이다.

• 과거형

☐ The patient gave consent for treatment.

환자가 치료받는 것을 허락하였다.

☐ Tylenol relieved her symptoms.

타이레놀이 그녀의 증세를 완화시켰다.

☐ The girl cried.

그녀는 울었다.

☐ I explained the procedure to the patient.

나는 환자에게 절차를 설명하였다.

☐ She questioned the course of treatment, and I explained.

그녀는 치료 과정에 대해 질문하였고 나는 설명을 하였다.

☐ The patient looked nervous and depressed.

환자는 긴장되고 우울해 보였다.

☐ She was being evasive in her answers.

그녀는 대답에 있어 회피적이었다.

☐ The patient looked pale.

환자가 창백해 보였다.

☐ The patient looked for a specialist.

환자는 전문의를 찾았다.

☐ Dr. Kim referred the patient to a colleague of his for treatment.

닥터 김은 환자를 치료를 위해 그의 동료에게 보냈다.

☐ He was brought to the clinic by one of his friend.

그는 그의 친구에 의해(의 도움으로) 이 병원에 왔다.

☐ I discussed with the patient his wanting to be sent back to home.

나는 환자와 그가 집으로 가고 싶다는 것에 대해 의논하였다.

☐ There were bilateral hands lesions.

양쪽 손에 병이 있다.

☐ Diastolic pressures were in the 110s.

수축기 혈압은 110 정도였다.

☐ She had multiple decubiti on her back.

그녀는 등에 다발성 욕창이 있었다.

☐ The specimen was sent to the pathology department.

표본물은 병리학과로 보내졌다.

☐ She was sent to the in-patient unit from the emergency room.

그녀는 응급실에서 입원실로 옮겨졌다.

☐ We requested a copy of her medical record.

우리는 그녀의 의료기록 1부를 요청했다.

☐ Doctor spoke to her mother.

의사는 그녀의 어머니와 이야기했다.

☐ At the time of discharge, he was told what to do.

퇴원할 때, 그는 무엇을 해야 하는지 들었다.

☐ She complained today of some recurring ulcers in her mouth.

그녀는 오늘 입안의 궤양이 재발했다고 호소했다.

☐ The patient clearly stated no allergies.

환자는 알레르기는 없다고 확실하게 말했다.

☐ The baby weighed 7 pounds 9 ounces.

아기의 몸무게는 7파운드 9온스이다.

• 과거 완료형

☐ She had finally completed her course of chemotherapy when I saw her in November.

그녀는 내가 11월에 만났을 때 (암의) 약물치료를 다 끝냈었다.

☐ He had had acute appendicitis 2 years ago.

그는 급성 충수염이 2년 전 발병했었다.

부사(Adverb)

☐ She breathe too slowly.

그녀는 너무 천천히 숨을 쉰다.

☐ The patient takes her medication faithfully.

환자는 정확하게 약을 복용하고 있다.

☐ The patient takes her medication too early.

환자는 약을 너무 일찍 먹었다.

☐ The patient brings her medication every time.

환자는 그녀의 약을 매번 가지고 온다.

☐ The patient barely remember what she had this morning.

환자는 오늘 아침 무엇을 먹었는지 거의 기억하지 못합니다.

☐ The patient records her blood sugar level daily.

환자는 매일 혈당치를 기록합니다.

☐ Physical therapy has been really helpful to release the symptoms.

물리치료는 증세를 완화시키는 데 매우 도움이 됩니다.

☐ He is not eating as often as he used to be.

그는 평소에 먹던 만큼 자주 먹지 않습니다.

☐ The patient is not complained with her foods.

환자는 음식에 대해 불평하지 않습니다.

☐ She has truly been a faithful patient.

그녀는 약속을 잘 지킵니다.

☐ The patient believes the medication has actually made him feel better.

환자는 약이 실제로 (증세가) 좋아지게 만든다고 믿습니다.

☐ She complained that her hair conditioner made her skin really sore.

그녀는 헤어 컨디셔너가 피부를 쓰리게 만든다고 불평하였습니다.

☐ She is doing very well after the procedure.

그녀는 처치 후에 잘 지내고 있습니다.

☐ He wakes up at night quite frequently to urinate.

그는 소변 보러 밤에 여러 번 일어납니다.

☐ Patient can walk only few minutes when she has short of breath.

환자는 숨이 가쁠 때 겨우 몇 분 정도만 걸을 수 있습니다.

☐ Doctor talked to the patient yesterday.

의사가 어제 환자에게 말했습니다.

☐ This newborn baby will be discharged tomorrow.

이 신생아는 내일 퇴원합니다.

☐ The nurse will call you on Friday.

간호사가 금요일에 전화를 드릴 것입니다.

전치사(Preposition)

☐ The patient is scheduled for a endoscopy.

환자는 내시경검사 예정이다.

☐ The sty on her left eye has been getting worse.

왼쪽 눈에 다래끼가 더 나빠졌습니다.

☐ Please wait until your name is called.

이름을 부를 때까지 기다리십시오.

☐ List your medicine on this patient form.

여기 환자 기록에 당신의 (복용하는) 약 이름을 다 기록하십시오.

☐ You should press here against your arm.

여기를 꾹 누르십시오.

접속사(Conjunction)

☐ Patient was told to bring her medicine and previous medical records.

환자는 약과 예전 의료기록을 가져오라는 말을 들었다.

☐ She can postpone her appointment until tomorrow or visit the clinic right now.

그녀는 약속을 내일까지 연기하든지 아니면 지금 의원을 방문할 수 있습니다.

☐ His headache is mild and intermittent.

그의 두통은 약하고 간헐적이다.

☐ The child or her mother were unable to explain the situation very well.

아이나 아이의 어머니나 상황을 잘 설명하지 못했다.

☐ The treatment will be beneficial not only for your muscle pain but also rheumatism.

치료는 근육통뿐 아니라 류머티즘에도 좋습니다.

☐ Do you know whether patient will stay tonight or not?

환자가 오늘 머물 건지 아닌지(입원상태) 아십니까?

☐ After arriving in the emergency room, the patient become conscious.

응급실에 도착한 후 환자는 의식이 돌아왔습니다.

☐ Patient left after his test is done.

환자는 검사가 끝난 후 돌아갔습니다.

문장의 이해

주어(Subject)와 술어(Predicate)로 이루어진다.

☐ The patient and her family + met with me at the emergency room.

주어 술어

환자와 그 가족은 나를 응급실에서 만났다.

☐ The course of treatment + has not determined yet.

치료 과정은 아직 결정되지 않았다.

• 단순 문장(Simple Sentence)

☐ The patient's past medical history is available.

환자의 과거 진료기록이 있습니다.

☐ Immediate treatment is critical to her prognosis.

그녀의 예후에 즉각적인 치료가 결정적으로 중요하다.

☐ Her family plan is to seek genetic counseling.

그녀 가족의 계획은 유전에 대한 상담(조언)을 해보려는 것이다.

☐ Her ampicillin and tylenol were started this morning.

그녀는 암피실린(항생물질)과 타이레놀(비피린계 진통 해열제)을 오늘 아침부터 복용하기 시작했다.

☐ He was given discharge instructions.

그에게 퇴원에 필요한 지시사항을 알려 주었다.

• 중문(Compound Sentence)

☐ The patient presented to ER with acute stomach pain, and ultrasound was significant for diagnosis.

환자는 응급실에 급성 복통으로 들어왔고, 초음파 검사는 진단을 위해 중요했다.

☐ The doctor explained the risks and benefits of the procedure, and the patient signed up the consent form for the surgery.

의사는 (의료적) 처치의 위험성과 이로운 점에 대해 설명했고, 환자는 수술을 위한 허락서에 서명을 하였다.

• 복합문장(Complex Sentence)

☐ The patient admitted to ER with chest pain, which had been chronic over the previous 2 hours.

환자는 가슴 통증으로 응급실에 들어왔고, 그 통증은 지난 2시간 동안 지속되었었다.

☐ ER team were not able to initiate the patient's pulse despite of aggressive resuscitation.

응급실 의료팀은 적극적인 소생술을 시도했음에도 불구하고 환자의 심장박동을 일으키지 못했다.

• 평서문(Declarative Sentence)

☐ She is well-educated and well developed female.

그녀는 훌륭한 교육을 받은(교양이 있는), (육체적으로) 잘 성장(발달)한 여성이다.

☐ Repeat urine cultures were ordered by the doctor.

의사가 소변 (박테리아 배양) 재검사를 요청했다.

• 완결문(Imperative Sentence)

☐ Please take these specimens to the nurse.

이 피검물을 간호사에게 가져가십시오.

☐ Try to hold tight my hand.

제 손을 꽉 잡아 보세요.

• 의문문(Interrogative Sentence)

☐ When was your last period?

마지막 월경이 언제였습니까?

☐ Are you allergic to Penicillin?

페니실린에 대해 알레르기 반응이 있으십니까!

• 감탄문(Exclamatory Sentence)

☐ His blood pressure come back to normal!

그의 혈압이 정상으로 돌아왔다!

☐ She delivered twin babies at 10:30 in the morning!

그녀는 아침 10시 30분에 쌍둥이를 출산하였다!

구두점의 정확한 사용(Punctuation)

• 문장의 마침표(Period)

문장의 마침을 표시하는 것 외에 의료기록에서 어떻게 마침표가 쓰이고 있는지 살펴보자.

• 소수점(Decimal Fraction)
- 6.665 mg
- 0.13 ml
- $15.95
- The urine specific gravity was 1.016. (소변의 비중)

• 약어: 약어에 쓰이는 구두점
- 퇴원기록(Discharge Note)의 예

☐ Elevate the arm for the next 24 hr.
24시간 동안 팔을 높이 올려놓으십시오.

☐ Take pain medicine q.4h. p.r.n.pain.
진통제를 4시간마다 통증이 있을 때 드십시오.

☐ Check body temperature t.i.d. for next 2 days.
이틀간 하루 세 번씩 체온을 재 보십시오.

☐ Follow up in Dr.'s office on Monday 24th of July.
7월 24일 진찰실에 재진을 하러 오십시오.

여기에서 의료기록에 흔하게 쓰이는 약어들을 살펴보자.

의료 약어의 예(Medical Abbreviations)

☐ A+A(awake and aware)	☐ 의식 있음
☐ aa(of each or ana)	☐ 각각, 각자, 혹은 같은 양
☐ ABG(arterial blood gas)	☐ 동맥혈 가스 분석법
☐ a.c.(before meals)	☐ 식사 전(ante cibum)
☐ ACU(ambulatory care unit)	☐ 외래통원
☐ AD(average day)	☐ 평일, 평상시
☐ ADL(activities of daily living)	☐ 일상 활동들
☐ ad lib(as desired)	☐ 임의로
☐ AFC(at earliest convenience)	☐ 조속히
☐ a.m.(before noon)	☐ 오전(ante meridiem)
☐ aq(water)	☐ 물

☐ ASAP(as soon as possible)	☐ 가능한 빨리
☐ p.m.(after noon)	☐ 오후(post meridiem)
☐ AP(anterior-posterior)	☐ 전엽, 후엽
☐ A & P(anterior and posterior)	☐ 전엽과 후엽
☐ ASA(aspirin)	☐ 아스피린(해열제)
☐ ASHD(arteriosclerosistic heart disease)	☐ 동맥 경화성 심장 질환
☐ AV(arteriovenous, atrioventricular)	☐ 동정맥의, (심장의) 방실 사이의
☐ b.i.d.(twice a day)	☐ 하루에 두 번(bis in die)
☐ BO(body odor)	☐ 체취
☐ bpm(beats per minute)	☐ 분당 박동수
☐ BS(bedside)	☐ 침상
☐ BS(breath sound)	☐ 숨소리
☐ BS(blood sugar)	☐ 혈당
☐ BS(bowel sound)	☐ 장명(장에서 나는 소리)
☐ BSC(beside care)	☐ 침상간호
☐ BSC(beside commode)	☐ 침상변기
☐ -c(with)	☐ ...과 함께
☐ CAD(coronary artery disease)	☐ 심장 동맥 질환
☐ CBC(complete blood count)	☐ 전혈구 계산치
☐ CHF(congestive heart failure)	☐ 울혈성 심부전
☐ cm(centimeter)	☐ 센티미터
☐ C/O(complains of)	☐ (고통 등) 불평, 호소
☐ C & S(culture and sensitivity)	☐ 배양 및 감수성 검사
☐ CSF(cerebrospinal fluid)	☐ 뇌척수액
☐ CT(computed tomography)	☐ 전산화단층조영술
☐ cu(cubic)	☐ 입방체의
☐ CVS(clean voided specimen)	☐ 배설물을 청소할 것
☐ CW(crutch walking)	☐ 목발
☐ DAT(diet as tolerated)	☐ 식사 잘함
☐ DIC(disseminated intravascular coagulation)	☐ 파종성혈관내응고

☐ DK(diet kitchen)	☐ 규정식
☐ DNR(do not resuscitate)	☐ 인공소생술 금지
☐ DOA(date of arrival) or (death on arrival)?	☐ 입원날짜 혹은 도착시 이미 사망
☐ DOB(date of birth)	☐ 생년월일
☐ Dx(diagnosis)	☐ 진단
☐ EBL(estimated blood loss)	☐ 추정 출혈량
☐ ECDB(encourage to cough and deep breathe)	☐ 기침유도와 심호흡
☐ ECF(extended care facility)	☐ 부차적 치료시설
☐ e.g.(for example)	☐ 예, 보기
☐ et al.(and other people)	☐ (이름들 뒤에서) 외(etalia)
☐ etc(and so forth)	☐ 등등
☐ Fe(iron)	☐ 철분
☐ FUO(fever of undetermined origin)	☐ 원인이 규명되지 않은 열
☐ g, gm(gram)	☐ 그램(무게)
☐ gr(grain)	☐ 곡물
☐ gtt(gtt drop, drops)	☐ (약학)방울
☐ Hb(hemoglobin or transcribed hemoglobin)	☐ 헤모글로빈
☐ HB(heart block)	☐ 심장 폐쇄
☐ Hct(hematocrit or transcribed hematocrit)	☐ 혈구를 혈장에서 분리하기 위한 원심 분리기
☐ HNV(has not voided)	☐ 소변 안 봄
☐ hs(at bedtime, hour of sleep)	☐ 수면할 때, 수면 시간
☐ HTN(hypertension)	☐ 고혈압
☐ Hx(history)	☐ 력, 역사
☐ i.e.(that is)	☐ 다시 말해서
☐ IM(intramuscular)	☐ 근육내의
☐ I & O(intake and output)	☐ 섭취와 배설
☐ IV(intravenous)	☐ 정맥 주사의
☐ kg(kilogram)	☐ 킬로그램
☐ KVO(keep vein open)	☐ 혈관 지속적 개방

- ☐ KUB(kidneys, ureters, and bladder) ☐ 신장, 수뇨관, 방광
- ☐ L(liter) ☐ 리터(액체의 양을 재는 단위)
- ☐ lb(pound) ☐ 파운드
- ☐ m(meter, minim) ☐ 미터
- ☐ mEq(milliequivalent) ☐ 밀리그램 당량
- ☐ mg(milligram) ☐ 밀리그램
- ☐ mcg(microgram) ☐ 마이크로그램(100만분의 1)
- ☐ ml(milliliter) ☐ 밀리리터(리터의 1000분의 1)
- ☐ mm(millimeter) ☐ 밀리미터(미터의 1000분의 1)
- ☐ NPO nothing by mouth ☐ 절식, 먹이지 말 것
- ☐ NS(normal saline) ☐ 생리 식염수
- ☐ NSAID(nonsteroidal anti inflammatory drugs) ☐ 비스테로이드성 항염증성 약들
- ☐ OTC(over the counter) ☐ 처방 없이 상점에서 구입이 가능한
- ☐ OU(each eye) ☐ 각각의 눈
- ☐ oz(ounce) ☐ 온스
- ☐ p.c.(after meals) ☐ 식후(post cibum)(약의 처방전 지시)
- ☐ PERRLA(pupils equal, round, reactive to light and accommodation) ☐ 동공의 빛과 (원근) 조절에 대한 동일한 반응
- ☐ P.O.(by mouth) ☐ 입으로, 경구적으로
- ☐ pp.(pages) ☐ 페이지
- ☐ p.r.n.(as needed whenever necessary) ☐ 필요할 때에
- ☐ q(every) ☐ 매번, 매회
- ☐ q.d.(every day) ☐ 매일
- ☐ q.6h.(every six hours) ☐ 매 6시간마다
- ☐ q.8h.(every eight hours) ☐ 매 8시간마다
- ☐ q.12h.(every twelve hours) ☐ 매 12시간마다
- ☐ qhr(every hour) ☐ 매 시간
- ☐ q.i.d.(four times a day) ☐ 하루 4회
- ☐ q2hr(every 2 hours) ☐ 매 2시간마다
- ☐ q.i.d.(four times a day) ☐ 하루 4회

☐ R/O(rule out)	☐ 배제, 제외
☐ ROM(range of motion)	☐ 관절 가동 범위
☐ Rx(prescription)	☐ 처방전
☐ s(without)	☐ ...없이
☐ subq(subcutaneous)	☐ 피하의
☐ SL(sublingual)	☐ 설하선, 혀밑의
☐ SOB(short of breath)	☐ 숨가쁨
☐ ss(one-half)	☐ 1/2 (2분의 1)
☐ stat(immediately)	☐ 즉시
☐ Sx(symptoms)	☐ 증상
☐ T & C(type and crossmatch)	☐ 유형과 교차적합
☐ t.i.d.(three times a day)	☐ 하루 3회
☐ TPR(temperature, pulse, respirations)	☐ 체온, 맥박, 호흡수
☐ TO(telephone order)	☐ 전화요청
☐ tsp(teaspoon)	☐ 티스푼(양)
☐ UA(urinalysis)	☐ 소변검사
☐ URI(upper respiratory infection)	☐ 상기도 감염
☐ UTI(urinary tract infection)	☐ 요로 감염
☐ VO(verbal order)	☐ 구두 주문
☐ WBC-(white blood count)	☐ 백혈구 수
☐ WNL(within normal limits)	☐ 정상치 내

* 참고: 복부의 위치에 대한 명칭

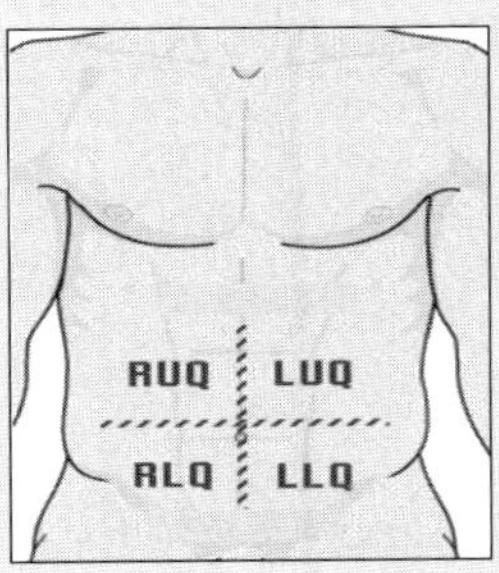

☐ LLQ(left lower quadrant)
(복부를 4등분 할 때) 왼쪽 아랫부분

☐ LUQ(left upper quadrant)
(복부를 4등분 할 때) 왼쪽 윗부분

☐ RUQ(right upper quadrant)
(복부를 4등분 할 때) 오른쪽 윗부분

☐ RLQ(right lower quadrant)
(복부를 4등분 할 때) 오른쪽 아랫부분

쉼표(Comma)

구두점 중에 가장 흔하게 쓰이는 것은 쉼표이다. 쉼표는 영어 문장에 있어 정확한 문장을 구사하는 데 꼭 필요한 도구가 되지만 또한 잘못 사용하면 문제를 일으킬 수 있는 소지를 갖고 있는 도구이기도 하다.

문장 속에서 쉼표가 어떻게 쓰이고 있는지 예문을 통해 살펴보자.

• 숫자

☐ Platelet count was 346,000.
혈소판 숫자는 34만 6천이다.

• 날짜

☐ The patient was last seen on April 28, 2011.
환자는 2011년 4월 28일 마지막으로 방문하였다.

☐ He had the surgery on July 10, 2007, at St. Vincent Hospital.
그는 성 빈센트 병원에서 2007년 7월 10일 수술을 받았다.

• 이름과 지위

☐ George A. Charles, MD
의사 찰스 조지 씨

☐ Mr. Campbell
캠벨 씨

☐ Howard Bush Jr.
하워드 부시 아들

☐ John D. Frank, DO(Doctor of Osteopathic Medicine)
의사(골장애 전문의) 프랭크 존 씨

• 유전자, 병명 표시

☐ The normal human karyotypes are 46, XX for female and 46, XY for male.
정상 여성 염색체 46 XX 남성 염색체 46 XY.

☐ E. coli

이콜라이균(대장균)

• 부수적인 구(Nonessential Clause) 혹은 단어(Nonessential Word)의 삽입

☐ Emily Parkins, who had a mammogram last year, came in for an examination today.

작년에 유방암 검사를 한, 에밀리 파킨스씨는 오늘 검진을 위해 방문했다.

☐ Please notice, if you will, date of the last health check up.

아시겠지만, 지난 건강 검진한 날을 주목해 주세요.

☐ We will get the opinion of Dr. Kwon, who has expertise in this area, prior to proceeding with surgery.

수술을 진행하기 전에 이 방면에 전문가인 닥터 권에게 의견을 구해야겠다.

☐ There is, no doubt, a reason for the sudden cardiac arrest.

틀림없이, 심장마비가 발생한 이유가 있을 것이다.

☐ Mrs. Lambert, Dr. Kim's patient, was admitted to Cancer Center yesterday.

닥터 김의 환자인, 램버트 부인은 암센터에 왔습니다.

☐ Ms. Lee, the head nurse, gave patient a copy of Dr.'s report.

수간호사인, 미스 리는 의사의 기록을 환자에게 주었다.

☐ John, the 37 yrs. old male patient, was admitted to ER today.

37세의 남성 환자인 존은, 오늘 응급실에 왔다.

☐ We will get the opinion of Dr. Shin, who has expertise in this area, prior to proceeding with surgery.

우리는 수술을 진행하기 전에 이 방면에 전문가인 닥터 신의 의견을 알아볼 것이다.

☐ This male patient presents today with her spouse, who drives the patient to his appointment.

이 남성 환자는 오늘, 그의 배우자가 차로 데리고 병원에 왔다.

• 삽입구

☐ This male patient should have, in my opinion, immediate surgery.

내 의견으로는 이 남성 환자는 즉시 수술을 해야만 한다.

☐ Her temperature, which has been high, fell suddenly now.

높았던 그녀의 체온이 이제 떨어졌다.

☐ Dr. Kwon is an expert, whether or not the patient care for his opinion, and I feel that you must follow his advice.

환자가 관심이 있든지 없든지 닥터 권은 전문가이고 나는 당신이 그의 충고를 따라야 한다고 생각합니다.

☐ All patients, wearing pacemakers, should be told to visit doctor for check up every 3 months.

맥박 조정기를 사용하고 있는 모든 환자는 3개월마다 검진을 위해 의사를 방문해야만 한다.

☐ She will, if possible, bring her previous medicine with her on her next visit.

그녀는, 가능하다면 다음 방문 때 전에 복용했던 약을 가져올 것이다.

• 도입구(Introductory Dependent Phrase, Clause)

☐ After the surgery was completed, he was transferred to ICU(Intensive Care Unit).

수술이 끝난 후에, 그는 중환자실로 옮겨졌다.

☐ Although she had been in pain for some time, she failed to seek medical attention.

그녀는 한동안 아팠지만, 의료적인 도움을 받지 못했다.

☐ When the patient is ready to leave, the wheel chair is ready to take him to the gate.

환자가 떠날 준비가 되었을 때, 그를 문까지 데려다 주기 위해 휠체어가 준비되었다.

☐ If you are not feeling better by tomorrow, do not hesitate to call Dr. Kim.

내일까지 좋아지지 않는다면, 망설이지 말고 닥터 김에게 전화하십시오.

☐ Only the second copy, which is a photo copy should be mailed to his primary doctor.

복사본, 즉 사진 복사본만 주치의에게 부쳐야 합니다.

☐ She used a walker in her both hands, but now she cannot use a walker at all because of pain in her wrists.

그녀는 두 손으로 보행기를 사용했었지만, 팔목의 통증으로 보행기를 전혀 사용할 수 없다.

• 문장의 전환

☐ The patient was given antibiotics for two days. Subsequently, she became more responsive.

환자에게 이틀 동안 항생제가 투여되었다. 그 결과로, 그녀는 좀 더 잘 반응할 수 있게 되었다.

☐ He was given Tylenol, however his headache did not improve.

그에게 타이레놀을 주었지만, 그의 두통은 나아지지 않았다.

☐ She was admitted to the emergency room after a major automobile accident. Despite of all efforts, we were unable to resuscitate her.

그녀는 큰 자동차 사고로 응급실에 들어왔다. 모든 노력에도 불구하고, 우리는 그를 소생시킬 수 없었다.

세미콜론, 콜론(Semi Colon, Colon)

• 세미콜론

☐ Doctor have requested to change his medication; The nurse have recorded.

의사는 그의 약을 바꾸라고 요청하였다; 간호사가 기록하였다.

☐ The nose is remarkable for terrible congestion; there is no discharge visible.

코에 심한 충혈(코막힘)이 두드러지게 나타난다; 분비물은 없다.

☐ Around the first of July, he developed pain in his chest, which he ignored for several days; and finally he saw me, at the request of his family doctor, on July 16.

7월 1일경, 그는 가슴에 통증을 느끼기 시작했으나 통증을 며칠 동안 (치료받지 않고) 방치했다; 그리고 그를 돌보는 가정의의 요청으로, 7월 16일 결국 나를 보러 왔다.

☐ There was no history of pneumonia, tuberculosis, chronic cough, or hemoptysis; and there was no exposure to substances at home, at work, or at school that may have contributed to this event.

폐렴, 결핵, 만성적 기침 혹은 객혈의 병력은 없었다; 그리고 집, 직장 혹은 학교에서 이런 종류의 증상을 일으킬 만한 어떤 유해물질에 노출된 적도 없었다.

☐ I attempted a labor induction with Pitocin, and contractions occurred; however, the patient failed to develop an effective labor pattern, and a doctor discharged her after six hours.

나는 피토신(자궁 수축제)으로 유도 분만을 시도했고 (산모의) 진통이 시작되었다; 그러나 환자는 효과적인 분만의 상태로 진전하는 데 실패하였고 의사는 6시간 후에 퇴원시켰다.

• 콜론

□ TEMPERATURE: 98.6F	□ 체온: 화씨 98.6도
□ PULSE: 70/min	□ 심박: 1분에 70회
□ RESPIRATIONS: 20/min	□ 호흡수: 1분에 20회
□ BLOOD PRESSURE: 130/70	□ 혈압: 130에 70 (수축기 혈압 130, 이완기 혈압 70)
□ Allergies: Allergic to AMOXICILLIN	□ 알레르기 반응: 아목시실린(항생제)에 대한 알레르기 반응
□ Allergies: No Known Allergies	□ 알레르기 반응: 알려진 알레르기 반응 없음
□ 2:00 p.m.	□ 오후 2시
□ Patient is scheduled to discharge at 4:30 p.m.	□ 환자는 오후 4시 30분에 퇴원하도록 예정되어 있다.
□ Cold agglutinins 1:4	□ 저온 응집율 1:4

□ Please bring the following items with you to the hospital: robe, slippers, toilet articles, and two pairs of pajamas.

다음 품목들을 소지하고 병원에 오십시오: 가운, 실내용 덧신, 세면용품, 잠옷 두 벌.

□ The following medications were suggested to the patient to alleviate her symptoms: Aspirin, Advil.

다음과 같은 약들이 환자에게 고통을 완화시키기 위해 권해졌습니다: 아스피린, 애드빌.

□ Doctor offered the patient several options for treatment: conservative observation, medical management, and surgical intervention.

의사는 몇 가지 치료를 환자에게 제안하였습니다. 조심스러운 관찰방법, 의료적 관리, 외과적 개입.

☐ Doctor see only one alternative: chemotherapy.
의사가 보는 단 한 가지 유일한 방법: 약물치료(암).

☐ We have one goal : fast relief from the pain.
우리의 한 가지 목표: 고통으로부터의 빠른 회복.

하이픈(-)과 사선(/)

• 하이픈(연자부호)

☐ anti-inflammatory	☐ 항염
☐ un-ionized	☐ 이온화하지 않은
☐ 10-to 12- year history	☐ 10～12년 (기간 동안의) 이력(내력)
☐ 3-to 4- inch incision	☐ 3～4인치 절개
☐ full-thickness graft	☐ 전층식피술
☐ split-thickness graft	☐ 분리층식피술
☐ figure-of-eight sutures	☐ 8자형 봉합
☐ 1st-, 2nd-, and 3rd-trimester symptom	☐ (임신기간 중) 처음 3개월, 두 번째 3개월, 세 번째 3개월
☐ re-treat(treat again)	☐ 재치료
☐ re-sign(sign again)	☐ 재서명
☐ re-collect(collect again)	☐ 재채집
☐ seizure-inducing drug	☐ 발작(을) 유도하는 약물
☐ end-to-end anastomosis	☐ (두 개의 관) 문합(술)
☐ ill-defined tumor mass	☐ (식별이) 불분명한 종양 덩어리
☐ non-Korean-speaking patient	☐ 한국말을 하지 못하는 환자
☐ AIDS-related complex	☐ 후천성면역결핍증과 관련된 문제
☐ behind-the-ear hearing aid	☐ 귀 뒤에 장착하는 보청기
☐ fat-soluble vitamins	☐ 지용성 비타민
☐ end-of-dose deterioration	☐ 약 사용 효과의 하락
☐ self-inflicted	☐ 자초한
☐ self-limited disease	☐ (병이) 한정된 과정을 겪는, 자체 한정적인

☐ ex-patient	☐ 과거 환자
☐ self-medicating	☐ 자가 치료적인
☐ an up-to-date medical history	☐ 현재까지의 의료(에 관계된) 내력
☐ a cause-and-effect relationship	☐ 원인과 결과의 관계
☐ an off-the-record comment	☐ 비공개를 전제로 하는 내용
☐ a well-developed female	☐ 잘 발달된(몸) 여성
☐ a fast-acting medication	☐ 속효성의 약
☐ second-floor inpatient unit	☐ 이층의(에 있는) 입원실
☐ random-access memory	☐ 임의 추출 기억 장치
☐ BP was 120-130 over 80-90	☐ 혈압(Blood Pressure)은 120-130에 80-90
☐ two 1-liter solutions	☐ 두 개의 1리터짜리 용액
☐ six 3-bed wards	☐ 6개의 3인실(3개의 침대가 있는) (입원)병동
☐ The Patient's father-in-law	☐ 환자의 장인 혹은 시아버지(배우자의 아버지)

☐ The patient was a 35-year-old female admitted with a history of chest pain.
환자는 가슴 통증의 병력을 가진 35세의 여성으로 병원에 들어왔다.

☐ The 50-year-old Caucasian female was admitted for shortness of breath and wheezing.
50세의 백인 여성은 숨가쁨과 쌕쌕거림의 증세로 병원에 들어왔다.

☐ She was admitted for right-sided chest pain.
그녀는 오른쪽 가슴 통증으로 병원에 들어왔다.

☐ The patient went for a chest x-ray.
환자는 가슴 엑스레이를 찍으러 갔다.

☐ She must go to her family physician for follow-up one week following her discharge.
그녀는 퇴원 일주일 후 재진을 위해 주치의에게 가야만 한다.

☐ The patient was evaluated for second-and-third degree burns to her right leg.
환자는 오른발에 2도 3도 화상을 입은 것으로 진단되었다.

☐ The patient was a well-developed 20-year-old female in no acute distress.
환자는 급성 통증이 없는 건강한 20세의 여성이었다.

☐ He is admitted with a 5-day fever.
그는 5일간의 열로 병원에 들어왔다.

☐ He is a 37-year-old, well-developed, well-balanced male.

그는 37세이고, 건강하고, 균형 잡힌 남성이다.

☐ I found the patient to be panic-stricken.

나는 환자가 공황 상태에 빠진 것을 알았다.

• 사선

☐ Date of admission: 02/13/2007 ☐ 입원일: 2007년 2월 13일

☐ Date of discharge: 02/25/2007 ☐ 퇴원일: 2007년 2월 25일

☐ She has 20/20 vision. ☐ 그녀는 20에 20 시력을 갖고 있다.

☐ His blood pressure is 110/80. ☐ 그는 혈압은 110에 80이다.

☐ The dosage is 150mg/day. ☐ 복용량은 하루에 150 밀리그램이다.

☐ Hemoglobin level was 14g/dL ☐ 헤모글로빈 수치 디시리터(diciliter)당 14 그램

g/dL이란 단위는 Albumin, Hemoglobin 등의 수치를 나타내는 데 쓰이는 단위이다.

☐ c/o: care of ☐ …에게 …씨 방(업무상 편지 수신인 이름 앞에 쓴다)

☐ 1-1/2 inch: one and half inch ☐ 1.5인치

☐ Her treatment/diagnostic planning was discussed with the caregiver.

그녀의 치료/진단 계획을 (환자, 여기서는 그녀) 돌보는 사람과 의논하였다.

☐ Doctor had a long discussion with patient's grandmother/legal guardian about the surgery.

의사는 환자의 할머니/법적 보호자와 긴 토론을 하였다.

• 숫자기록

의료기록에 등장하게 되는 수의 명시에는 여러 가지가 있다.

☐ 4-0 silk(suture) ☐ 실크 봉합사 사이즈 4-0 (0.7 metric)

☐ 2-0 chromic suture ☐ 크롬 봉합사 2-0

☐ #16 FR catheter ☐ (요도, 혈관 등에 삽입하는) 도관(카테터) 사이즈 16 FR(1FR = 0.33mm)

☐ Cranial nerves II-XII were intact. ☐ 뇌신경 II-XII는 손상되지 않았다(건강하다).

- ☐ The patient has a 4 cm stage I decubitus ulcer.
  ☐ 환자는 4센티미터 크기, 1단계 욕창성 궤양을 갖고 있다.
- ☐ The patient has 2+ edema in her right ankle.
  ☐ 환자는 오른쪽 무릎에 2+ 수종이 있다.
- ☐ Vision is 20/20 in the right eye.
  ☐ 오른쪽 눈 시력이 20/20이다.
- ☐ Tylenol #3 q.6h. p.r.n. for pain
  ☐ Tylenol #3 6시간마다 필요할 때 통증에 복용할 것
- ☐ The exact size of an area, growth or mass is transcribed for example: The decubitus 2×4 cm ulcer measured 2×4 cm.
  ☐ 부위, 발병 변화, 매스의 정확한 크기를 예(보기)로 기록하였다: 욕창성 위궤양 크기로 측정되었다.
- ☐ The sponge count was correct×2.
  ☐ 스폰지 숫자 확인하였다. 두 번 확인.
- ☐ 2-1/2 inches
  ☐ 2.5인치
- ☐ 3-3/4 hours
  ☐ 3시간 45분
- ☐ three-fourths of the bottle
  ☐ 4분의 3 병
- ☐ two-thirds of area
  ☐ 3분의 2 범위
- ☐ The initial consultation is $125.00.
  ☐ 첫 번째 상담은 125불이다.

괄호(Brackets)의 사용

☐ The patient had had multiple complaints(nausea, vomiting, fever, intermittent headache).
환자는 여러 가지 통증을 갖고 있다(매슥거림, 구토, 발열, 간헐적인 두통).

☐ A great deal of swelling was present(more so on the right than the left).
상당한 부종이 나타났다(왼쪽보다 오른쪽이 더 심하다).

☐ This male infant is improving(despite his slight fever) and we plan to discharge him by tomorrow.
이 남자아이는 상태가 호전되었고(약간의 열은 있지만) 우리는 내일 퇴원시킬 예정이다.

☐ We started her on (pain medicine, antibiotic) seems to be doing an adequate job of recovering from the surgery.
우리는 그녀에게 (진통제와 항생제) 투여를 시작했고 수술 후 회복에 적합한 방법처럼

보인다.

☐ He has a long history of known diagnosis, including (1) chronic arthritis (2) osteoporosis (3) cardiovascular disease.

그는 오래된 (1) 만성 관절염 (2) 골다공증 (3) 심근계 질병의 증세를 갖고 있다.

☐ [HCO3-]

화학 농도 표시 하이드로겐 카보네이트(hydrogen carbonate)

진료 기록 시 알아두어야 할 용어(Medical Transcription Terms)

• 여러 가지 의학문 명칭(Terms for Specialist)

☐ Cardiology	☐ 심장병학, 심장학
☐ Dermatology	☐ 피부과학
☐ Gastroenterology	☐ 위장병학
☐ Hematology	☐ 혈액학
☐ Immunology	☐ 면역학
☐ Nephrology	☐ 신장학
☐ Neurology	☐ 신경학
☐ Obstetrics and Gynecology	☐ 산부인과학
☐ Oncology	☐ 종양학
☐ Ophthalmology	☐ 안과학
☐ Orthopedics	☐ 정형외과학
☐ Otorhinolaryngology	☐ 이비인후과학
☐ Psychiatry	☐ 정신과학
☐ Pulmonology	☐ 호흡기학
☐ Urology	☐ 비뇨기과학

• 흔하게 쓰이는 의료 용어들

☐ Ablation ☐ 1. 절제, 제거 2. 차단

Removing a part of the body through surgery

☐ Acampsia ☐ 관절강직

Inability to bend or extend a joint

☐ Acroagnosis ☐ 팔다리인식불능(증), 사지실인증

Lack of sensation in an arm or leg

☐ Acronesthesia ☐ 지단 무감각

Loss of sensation in one or more limbs

☐ Acrotic Pulse ☐ 무맥박-, 약한 맥박-

A very weak pulse

☐ Actinocymography ☐ 엑스선 활동 조영술

X-raying an organ while it is moving

☐ Afebrile ☐ 무열성(無熱性)의

Without fever, person whose temperature is normal

☐ Aglutition ☐ 삼킴불능(증)

Difficulty in swallowing

☐ Algesic ☐ 통각의

Painful

☐ Ambulatory ☐ 보행의

Able to walk by oneself

☐ Amputation ☐ 1. 절단, 자름 2. 절단술

Removal of a limb or part of a limb through surgery

☐ Analgesia ☐ 1. 진통 2. 무통증

Absence of pain in response to stimulation that is normally painful

☐ Analgesic Drugs ☐ 진통제

Pain-relieving medications(anodynes)

☐ Anemia ☐ 빈혈

Insufficiency of red blood cells, either in quality or quantity

☐ Anesthesia ☐ 마취, 무감각

Loss of sensation; usually produced for a painless surgery

☐ Angina Pectoris ☐ 협심증, 가슴조임증

Pain in the chest, sometimes radiating to the left arm, caused by a spasm of the coronary artery of the heart

☐ Ankylosis ☐ 관절굳음증, 강직

Stiffening or fixation of a joint

☐ Antagonist ☐ 1. 대항제, 길항제 2. 대항근

A drug which neutralizes the effect of another drug

☐ Anti-Inflammatory Drugs ☐ 진통제, 해열제 및 항염제

Medication for reducing inflammation

☐ Aphasia ☐ 〈병리〉 실어증(失語症)

Difficulty with speech and ability to communicate

☐ Appendectomy ☐ 〈외과〉 충수(蟲垂: 맹장) 절제(술)

Removal of the appendix by surgery

☐ Apnea ☐ 무호흡

A temporary stopping of breathing, often occurring during sleep

☐ Atrophy ☐ 〈병리〉 (영양 부족 따위에 의한) 위축증, 소모증

The size decreases, or wasting away

☐ Benign ☐ 양성(암이 아닌)

Not malignant(not cancerous)

☐ Carcinoma ☐ 〈병리〉 암(cancer), 악성 종양

A malignant growth(cancerous)

☐ Catheter ☐ 카테터, 도관, 도자

A hollow tube for passage into a structure, to inject or remove fluid or blood

☐ Central Pain ☐ 중추성 통증

Pain associated with a lesion of the central nervous system

☐ Central Venous Catheter ☐ 중심 정맥 카테터

A hollow plastic tube inserted into a vein in the arm or neck, and pushed forward until it reaches the vena cava in the chest

☐ Contracture ☐ 구축, 연축

The shortening of a muscle, tendon or other structure resulting in inability to straighten or flex and extend

☐ Cryesthesia ☐ 한랭과민증

Sensitivity to cold

☐ Dementia ☐ 치매

Loss of mental capacity

☐ Denervate ☐ 탈신경

To cut a nerve going to or from an organ or structure, mainly to relieve pain

☐ Diabetes mellitus ☐ 당뇨병

A metabolic disorder that produces hyperglycemia(increased blood sugar). Common symptoms may be increased thirst, increased urination and loss of weight

☐ Diastolic Pressure ☐ 확장기압

The blood pressure level when the heart muscle is relaxed

☐ Dorsal ☐ 1. 등쪽의-, 등의- 2. 후방의-

Refers to the back, opposite of ventral

☐ Dorsum ☐ 1. 등, 뒤 2. 등쪽, 후방

The back of an organ or body part

☐ Dysesthesia ☐ 1. 이상감각 2. 불쾌감각

An unpleasant abnormal sensation, whether spontaneous or evoked

☐ Dysphagia ☐ 〈병리〉 연하(嚥下) 곤란

difficult to swallow

☐ Dystrophy ☐ 근육퇴행위축

Abnormal development, progressive changes, and degeneration that may result from defective nutrition of tissue

☐ Echocardiography ☐ 심장초음파검사

A test in which sound waves are directed at the heart to get information on the health of the heart muscles and heart function

☐ Edema ☐ 부종

Excessive accumulation of fluid in the body tissue leading to swelling

☐ Endocrine ☐ 〈생리〉 내분비선; 내분비물, 호르몬(또는 endocrinal, endocrinic, endocrinous) 내분비(선, 물)의

Refers to glands in the body that secrete hormones into the bloodstream

Examples: pituitary, thyroid, and adrenals

☐ Electrocardiography ☐ 심전도검사

The recording of the electrical impulses of the heart(EKG, ECG)

☐ Electroencephalography ☐ 뇌파검사, 뇌전도검사

The recording of brain waves(EEG)

☐ Electromyograph ☐ 근전도검사기

An instrument which records the electrical impulses that pass through a muscle as it contracts and relaxes(EMG)

☐ Endoscope ☐ 내시경

An instrument used to look into body cavities and openings

☐ Erythema ☐ 홍반

A patch of redness of the skin

☐ Exacerbation ☐ 악화, 증진(增進), 증악(增惡)

Flare-up or relapse of a condition or disease

☐ Fascia ☐ 근막

Connective tissue located in various places throughout the body

☐ Febrile ☐ 열성경련, 열성발작

Feverish; relating to an elevation in body temperature above 98.6° F

☐ Fibrosis ☐ 섬유증, 섬유화

Thickening and scarring of connective tissue which replaces the normal components of a structure

☐ Fluoroscopy ☐ 투시검사

X-Raying a part of the body and recording the rays on the fluorescent screen to view various organs in motion

☐ Ganglion Cyst ☐ 결절종

A cyst of the sheath of a tendon, frequently appearing about the wrist

☐ Glucose ☐ 〈생화학〉 글루코오스, 포도당; 물엿(starch syrup)

sugar, or blood sugar.

☐ Gout ☐ 통풍

A type of arthritis or inflammation in a joint caused by excess uric acid in the blood

☐ Hematemesis ☐ 토혈, 혈액구토

Vomiting of blood

☐ Hydrosis ☐ 발한 과다증, 다한증

Excessive perspiration

☐ Hypalgesia ☐ 통각감퇴

Decreased sensation to pain

☐ Hyperasthesia ☐ 지각과민

Over-sensitivity to touch and light pressure

☐ Hyperesthesia ☐ 감각과민(증)

Excess sensitivity, such as to touch or pinprick

☐ Hyperglycemia ☐ 고혈당(증)

Excessive sugar in the blood

☐ Hyperhydrosis ☐ 땀과다증, 다한증

Excessive sweating

☐ Hyperpiesis ☐ 이상 고혈압증, 이상 고압

High blood pressure; hypertension

☐ Hyperpnea ☐ 과다호흡, 호흡항진

Rapid and exceptionally deep breathing

☐ Hyperpyrexia ☐ 1. 고열(증) 2. 열요법

High fever

☐ Hypertension ☐ 고혈압

High blood pressure

☐ Hypesthesia ☐ 감각저하

Decreased sensitivity, as lessened appreciation of the sense of pain or touch

☐ Hypoalgesia ☐ 통각감퇴(痛覺減退)

Diminished sensitivity to noxious stimulation

☐ Hypoesthesia ☐ 감각저하

Diminished sensitivity to stimulation, excluding special senses

☐ Hypoglicemia ☐ 〈병리〉 저혈당(低血糖)(증)

Too little sugar in the blood

☐ Hyporeflexia ☐ 반사저하, 반사감퇴

Diminished reflexes

☐ Hypotension ☐ 저혈압

Low blood pressure

☐ Incision ☐ 〈의학〉 (외과의) 절개

A cut usually made for surgery reasons

☐ Indwelling catheter ☐ 유치카테터, 유치도관

One that is left in place for prolonged periods of time

☐ Lancinating Pain ☐ 칼로 베는 통증, 난자통

A shooting, knife-like, sudden, severe pain

☐ Lateral ☐ 가쪽-, 외측-

Refers to the side

☐ Lightening Pain ☐ 전격통(증)

Severe, sharp pains caused by nerve irritation

☐ Magnetic Resonance Imagining (MRI) ☐ 핵자기공명영상법(단층 촬영법)

A technique for viewing internal organs and bones; and for creating many of the images formerly revealed only by X-rays

☐ Minimally Invasive Surgery ☐ 최소침습수술

Operations performed through an endoscope or laparoscope, using the smallest incisions, some no more than approximately two-thirds of an inch in diameter

☐ Multiple Sclerosis ☐ 다발경화증

A chronic disease of the nervous system leading to partial paralysis, changes in speech, inability to walk, etc.

☐ Myoclonus ☐ 간대성근경련(증)

Abnormal muscle twitching

☐ Myomalacia ☐ 근(육)연화증, 근(육)무름증

Degeneration of muscle

☐ Myositis ☐ 근(육)염

Inflammation of muscle

☐ Myotonia ☐ 근(육)긴장증

Spasm of muscle

☐ Neonatal ☐ 신생아

Relating to or affecting the infant during the first month after birth

☐ Neuritis ☐ 신경염

An inflammatory or degenerative condition of a nerve

☐ Osteoarthritis ☐ 골관절염

A form of arthritis associated with bone and cartilage degeneration; seen mostly in aging people

☐ Osteochodritis ☐ 골연골염, 골연골염

Inflammation of a bone and cartilage

☐ Osteodynia ☐ 골통증

Pain in a bone

☐ Osteoporosis ☐ 골다공증

A loss in bony substances producing brittleness and softness of bones; often seen in aging people or those with debility (weakness)

☐ Pain threshold ☐ 동통역치(疼通閾値). 인식할 수 있는 통증의 가장 작은 경험

The point at which one feels pain. A person with a low pain threshold feels pain sooner than one with a high threshold

☐ Pituitary ☐ 〈해부〉= ~ body[gland]. 뇌하수체의(뇌하수체 호르몬의 과잉 분비에 의한), 말단 비대의

The master endocrine gland that secretes hormones that control growth and reproduction. Examples: growth hormone, prolactin, and adrenocorticotropic hormone, etc.

☐ Polyarthritis ☐ 다발성관절염

Inflammation of several joints

☐ Polymyositis ☐ 다발성근육염

Inflammation of several groups of muscles

☐ Radiculopathy ☐ 신경뿌리병(증), 신경근병(증)

Disease of the spinal nerves

☐ Rales ☐ 수포음(水泡音), 나음

An abnormal sound heard accompanying the normal respiratory sounds on auscultation of the chest

☐ Rebound Reaction ☐ 반향반감

A flare-up of symptoms when medication is abruptly terminated

☐ Referred Pain ☐ 연관통증

Pain which is felt some distance from the site of its origin

☐ Reflex ☐ 반사

An uncontrollable (involuntary) response to a particular stimulation

light reflex 빛반사 patellar reflex 무릎반사

☐ Reflux ☐ 역류

Flowing in a backward direction, as the flowing of the intestinal contents back to the stomach

☐ Remission ☐ 1. 완화 2. 진정

A clearing up of a disease or its symptoms

☐ Rhizotomy ☐ 신경뿌리절단(술), 신경근절단(술)

Surgery to cut the roots of spinal nerves, carried out to relieve incurable pain

☐ Romberg Test ☐ 롬버그 테스트

A test used by doctors in a neurological examination(to keep one's balance when standing with eyes closed)

☐ Spasm ☐ 〈의학〉 경련, 쥐(convulsion), 긴장성 경련

An abrupt and forceful contraction of a muscle usually associated with marked pain or discomfort

☐ Subcutaneous ☐ 피하조직(피부에서 진피의 아랫부분)

Underneath the skin

☐ Sudeck's Atrophy ☐ 수데크 위축병(Sudeck: 독일의 외과의사)

Degeneration of bone following an injury

☐ Sudomotor Changes ☐ 땀샘운동성-, 한선운동성 변화

Increased or decreased sweating

☐ Sympathectomy ☐ 교감신경절제(술)

Removal of some of the sympathetic nerves

☐ Symptoms ☐ 증세, 증상

Objective outward signs of an illness

☐ Syndrome ☐ 〈병리〉 증후군

A group of symptoms

☐ Syncope ☐ 실신

Fainting

☐ Systolic Blood Pressure ☐ 수축기혈압

The force with which blood is pumped when the heart muscle is contracting

☐ Telagia ☐ 연관통증

Pain radiating to another part of the body; referred pain

☐ Thyroid ☐ 〈해부〉 갑상선의, 갑상선; 갑상 연골; 갑상선 동맥[정맥]; 〈약학〉 갑상선제(劑)

An endocrine gland in the neck that produces hormones that help regulate metabolism

☐ Tonsillectomy ☐ 〈외과〉 편도(선) 절제[적출](술)

Removal of the tonsils by a surgical procedure

☐ Ultrasound ☐ 1. 초음파 2. 초음파촬영(술)

A type of imaging technique which uses high-frequency sound waves

• 의료기록자가 사용하는 줄임말

☐ adls(activities of daily living) ☐ 일상생활능력

☐ bec(because) ☐ 왜냐하면

☐ ch.stick(chapstick) ☐ 입술크림(입술 튼 데 바르는)

☐ diff(difficult) ☐ 어렵다

☐ exer(exercise) ☐ 운동

☐ fibj(fibrillation) ☐ 잔떨림

☐ glip(glipizide) ☐ 글리피지드(약)

☐ hpi(history of present illness) ☐ 현병력

☐ imm(immediate) ☐ 즉각의, 즉각적인

☐ jvd(jugular venous distention) ☐ 경정맥 팽만

☐ kin(kinesis) ☐ 1. 운동성 2. 운동력변형

☐ laby(laboratory) ☐ 검사실

- ☐ metab(metabolism) ☐ 대사
- ☐ nec(necessary) ☐ 필요한
- ☐ ocad(obstructive coronary artery disease) ☐ 폐쇄 관상 동맥질환
- ☐ palps(palpitations) ☐ 두근거림
- ☐ ques(question) ☐ 질문
- ☐ radj(radiation) ☐ 방사선
- ☐ satj(satisfaction) ☐ 만족
- ☐ testo(testosterone) ☐ 테스토스테론
- ☐ uw(underwent) ☐ 받았다
- ☐ verr(verrucous) ☐ 사마귀 모양
- ☐ w(we) ☐ 우리
- ☐ xfer(transfer) ☐ 옮기다, 전이하다
- ☐ yr(year) ☐ 한해
- ☐ zoc(zocor) ☐ 조코(약)

• 진단을 위한 검사(Diagnostic Test)의 종류

- ☐ Anoscopy ☐ 항문경 검사(법)
- ☐ Arthroscopy ☐ 관절경 검사(법)
- ☐ Barium Tests ☐ 바리움 소화기 검사
- ☐ Blood Tests ☐ 혈액 검사
- ☐ Bone Density Test ☐ 골밀도 검사
- ☐ Bone Marrow Biopsy Test ☐ 생척수체 검사
- ☐ Bone Scan ☐ 골주사 검사
- ☐ Bronchoscopy ☐ 기관지경술
- ☐ CAT Scan ☐ 컴퓨터X선체축 단층사진
- ☐ CT Scan(Computed Tomography) ☐ 컴퓨터 단층 촬영
- ☐ Colonoscopy ☐ 검사장내시경
- ☐ Cystoscopy ☐ 방광경 검사
- ☐ Echocardiogram ☐ 심(장)초음파상
- ☐ EEG - electroencephalogram ☐ 뇌파 검사

☐ EKG - electrocardiogram	☐ 심전도 검사
☐ Electrocardiography	☐ 심전도법
☐ Endoscopy	☐ 내시경술
☐ Endometrial Biopsy	☐ 자궁내막 생검
☐ Exercise Stress Test	☐ 운동부하 검사
☐ Flow Cytometry	☐ 유세포 측정기
☐ FOB(Fecal Occult Blood Test)	☐ 대변잠혈 검사
☐ Genetic Testing	☐ 유전자 검사
☐ HIV Tests	☐ 에이즈 검사
☐ Hysteroscopy	☐ 자궁경 검사
☐ Intravenous Pyelogram(IVP)	☐ 정맥신우조영사진
☐ Kidney-Ureter-Bladder(KUB) Radiography	☐ 신장요관방광 방사선촬영
☐ Laparoscopy	☐ 복강경 검사
☐ Liver Function Tests	☐ 간기능 검사
☐ Lymph node Biopsy Test	☐ 림프관 생검
☐ Mammography	☐ 유방암 검사
☐ Mediastinoscopy	☐ 종격내시경
☐ MRI	☐ 자기 공명 영상
☐ Myelography	☐ 척수조영(술)
☐ Oxygen Saturation Test	☐ 산소포화도 심사
☐ PET Scan	☐ 양자방출 단층촬영
☐ Pap Smear	☐ 자궁암 검사
☐ PSA(Prostate Specific Antigen)	☐ 전립선 특이 항원
☐ Pulmonary Function Test	☐ 폐기능 검사
☐ Renal Function Tests	☐ 신장기능 검사
☐ Radioimmunoassay	☐ 방사면역측정법
☐ Rapid Strep Test	☐ 신속 항원 검사
☐ Scratch Test for Allergies	☐ 피부 알레르기 테스트
☐ Sigmoidoscopy	☐ 구불창자 내시경 검사
☐ Skin Biopsy	☐ 피부 생검

☐ Tonometry ☐ 촉진안압측정

☐ Ultrasound ☐ 초음파 검사

☐ Urinalysis ☐ 요검사

☐ X-ray ☐ 엑스레이

3) 환자 의료기록

Chart Note ① Internal Medicine 내과 한글본

내과

환자 이름
생년월일: 05/15/48

03/14/01(진료일자)
(환자)는 오늘 종합 검진을 위해 내원하였다. 환자의 과거 의료, 수술내력, 사회적, 가족적 배경의 내용을 최근의 정보로 수정하였다. 환자의 지난 2주~2주 반 정도의 기간에 나타난 감기, 독감 같은 병력에 대한 기관별 검사는 주목할 만하다. 그녀는 분비물은 없으나 기침을 한다. 그녀는 안면통이나 치통은 없다. 그녀는 색이 있는 콧물도 없다. 그녀는 열이나 오한도 없다. 그녀는 설사를 했다. 그녀는 한 번 구토를 하였다. 그녀는 계속해서 기침을 해서 흉통을 느낀다. 그녀는 오늘 코흘림이 좀 호전되었다고 한다. 이 외에 기관별 검사는 모두 정상이다.

신체검사:

생체: 키 6피트 $3\frac{1}{2}$인치. 몸무게는 178파운드, 7파운드 감량됨. 맥박 60. 혈압 106/72.

피부: 의심되는 병변 없음.

머리, 눈, 귀, 코, 목구멍: 눈동자 동일하고 빛에 반응, 외안근 움직임 정상, 형광투시경 검사는 추간판에 출혈이나 삼출물 소견은 없다. 기관지는 깨끗하다. 고막은 정상이다.

목: 임파선 갑상선 병변 또는 이상음 없음.

가슴: 폐는 청진기로 들어 보았을 때와 타진 결과 깨끗함.

심장: S3, S4 없이 S1과 S2는 정상. 심잡음 없음.

* 심전도(ECG:electrocardiogram) 검사결과 그래프 상에 S-wave에 대한 소견이다.

유방: 덩어리나 분비물 없음. 겨드랑이 임파선 이상 발견된 바 없음.

복부: 대장음 활발(정상). 간 비장비대, 압통 또는 덩어리 발견된 바 없음. 외부생식기 정상. 자궁과 자궁경부 적출 수술로 소실. 손으로 하는 검사결과 덩어리 없음.

직장질: 확인함.

사지: 곤봉증, 청색증 혹은 부종 없음. 맥박은 2+ 이상음 없음.

신경계: 병소 없음.

결절: 림프절병 발병.

검사: 검사결과는 기다리고 있고 전화가 올 것이다.

다음 페이지 2에서 계속......

Chart Note ① Internal Medicine 내과 영문본

Internal Medicine

Patient Name
DOB: 05/15/48

03/14/01
Jane presents today for comprehensive evaluation. The patient's past medical, surgical, social history, and family history should be as per updated front face sheet. The patient's review of systems is remarkable for a history of cold and flu-like illness that has been present for the last two to two and a half weeks. She has had a cough that has been nonproductive. She has had no facial or tooth pain. She has noted no colored nasal drainage. She has had no fevers or chills. She has had some loose bowel movements. She has had one emesis. She states she continues to have cough. Her chest feels sore because of all the coughing. She states her runny nose has diminished somewhat today. Review of systems is otherwise negative.

PHYSICAL EXAMINATION:

VITALS: Height 6ft 3-1/2". Weight is 178 pounds, which is down 7 pounds. Pulse 60. Blood pressure 106/72.

SKIN: No suspicious lesions.

HEENT: Pupils are equal and reactive to light. The extraocular movements are intact. Fluoroscopic exam shows the discs to be flat and without hemorrhages or exudates. The pharynx is clear. Tympanic membranes are normal.

NECK: No adenopathy, thyromegaly, or bruits.

CHEST: Lungs are clear to auscultation and percussion.

CARDIAC: Examination shows normal S1 and S2 without S3, S4, or murmur.

BREASTS: No masses or discharge. No axillary adenopathy is noted.

ABDOMEN: Bowel sounds are active. No hepatosplenomegaly, tenderness, or masses are noted. Normal external genitalia. Uterus and cervix are surgically absent. Bimanual exam shows no masses.

RECTOVAGINAL: Confirmed.

EXTREMITIES: No clubbing, cyanosis, or edema. Pulses are 2+ and full without bruits.

NEUROLOGIC: Nonfocal.

NODES: No lymphadenopathy is noted.

LABS: Laboratory studies are pending and will be called.

continued page 2......

Chart Note ① Internal Medicine 내과 한글본

내과

평가:

1. 건강검진
2. 골반 검사와 자궁암 검사
3. 전조 증상 없는 편두통
4. 급성 상기도 감염
5. 고지혈증

계획:

환자에게 검사결과를 알려준다. 환자(그녀)는 6개월 후 여기에서 다시 검진할 것이다. 그때 지방질 검사를 재검사할 것이다.

환자(그녀)는 열, 오한, 가래가 나오는 기침 혹은 색이 있는(투명하지 않은) 부비강 분비물이 있을 경우에는 전화를 할 것이다.

결과를 기다리고 있는 검사: 혈액 검사, 소변 검사, 기본 검사, 지질 검사, 대변 잠혈검사

검사/진단에 의한 요청: 6개월 내에 지질 검사

다음 예약: 6개월 내에 재진

Chart Note ① Internal Medicine 내과 영문본

Internal Medicine

ASSESSMENT:

1. Health maintenance exam
2. Pelvic exam and Pap smear
3. Migraine headache without aura
4. Acute URI
5. Hyperlipidemia

PLAN:

Will advise the patient of her laboratory results. She will follow up here in six months. Will recheck her lipids at that time. Patient will call if she develops any fevers, chills, productive cough or colored sinus drainage.

PENDING LABS: Hemogram, urinalysis, basic, lipids, stool for Hemoccult
LABS/DIAGNOSTIC ORDERS: Lipids in six months

NEXT APPOINTMENT: Follow up in six months

단어 정리

□ comprehensive	□ 포괄적인, 모든 것을 포함하는; 광범위한
□ evaluation	□ (의학상의) 평가, 감정
□ medical history	□ 병력
□ surgical history	□ 외과적 수술 내력
□ social history	□ 사회력, 사회적 배경
□ family history	□ 가족력
□ cold	□ 감기
□ flu-like illness	□ 독감 같은 병
□ cough	□ 기침
□ nonproductive	□ (기침이) 마른, 가래·담을 수반하지 않는
□ colored nasal drainage	□ 색이 있는 콧물
□ fever	□ 열, 발열
□ chill	□ 오한
□ loose bowel movements	□ 무른 변(loose stool) 잦은 배설, 설사(frequent bowel movement)
□ review of systems	□ 기관별 검진
□ vitals(vital sign)	□ 생체, 활력 징후(vital sign: 체온, 혈압, 맥박, 호흡수)
□ height	□ 키
□ weight	□ 몸무게, 체중
□ pulse	□ 맥박
□ blood pressure	□ 혈압
□ lesion	□ 〈병리〉 (조직·기능의) 장애, 병소(病巢); 병변(病變)
□ HEENT(Head, Eye, Ear, Nose, Throat)	□ 머리, 눈, 귀, 코, 목
□ pupil	□ 〈해부〉 눈동자, 동공(瞳孔)
□ extraocular	□ 〈해부〉 외안근(外眼筋)
□ intact	□ 변하지 않은; 원래대로의, 건전(완전)한; 상처 없는
□ Funduscopic(dilated funduscopic examination)	□ 확장안저검사
□ hemorrhage	□ 〈병리〉 출혈

□ exudate	□ 삼출(滲出); 삼출물(액)
□ pharynx	□ 〈해부〉 인두
□ tympanic	□ 〈해부·동물〉 중이(귀)의
□ mebrane	□ (동·식물 조직의) 막, 얇은 막, 피막(皮膜); 막조직
□ adenopathy	□ 샘병(증), 선병(증)
□ thyromegaly (abnormally enlarged thyroid gland)	□ 갑상선 비대증
□ bruits	□ 〈의학〉 (청진기로 들을 수 있는) 이상음
□ auscultation	□ 〈의학〉 청진(법)
□ percussion	□ 〈의학〉 타진(법)
□ murmur(heart murmur)	□ 〈의학〉 심장 잡음(雜音)
□ mass	□ 종괴
□ discharge	□ 분비물
□ axillary	□ 겨드랑이의
□ hepatosplenomegaly	□ 간지라 비대, 간비장 비대
□ tenderness	□ 압통, 누름통증
□ genitalia	□ 〈해부〉 생식기, 성기; 외음부(外陰部)
□ uterus	□ 〈해부·동물〉 자궁(womb)
□ cervix	□ 〈해부〉 경부(頸部), 목 (자궁·방광 따위의) 경상부(頸狀部)
□ bimanual	□ 두 손으로 하는, 두 손을 필요로 하는
□ clubbing, digital clubbing	□ 손가락곤봉증, 발가락곤봉증
□ cyanosis	□ 〈병리〉 치아노오제, 청색증(靑色症)
□ edema	□ 〈병리〉 부종(浮腫), 수종 (또는 oedema)
□ nonfocal	□ 〈병리〉 병소(病巢)가 없는, 소상(巢狀)이 아닌
□ nodes(lymph nodes)	□ 림프절
□ lymphadenopathy	□ 림프절병(증)
□ rectovaginal	□ 직장질-, 곧창자질-
□ URI(Upper Respiratory Infection)	□ 상기도 감염
□ hemogram	□ 혈액상(血液像), 헤모그램
□ urinalysis	□ 소변 검사(분석). (또는 uranalysis)
□ lipids	□ 〈생화학〉 지방질[지방·납(蠟)·유(類)지방질의 총칭]
□ hemoccult test	□ 잠혈검사

Chart Note ② Endocrinology 내분비학과 한글본

내분비학과

추천해 준 의사: Dr. Richard Hann
주요증상: 갑상선 결절

현 병력:
페트리샤는 53세 여성으로, 상당히 심한 머리의 불쾌감과 통증을 갖고 있다. 머리의 MRI에서는 C5와 C6에 퇴행성 변화와 척수의 압박과 함께 추간판의 돌출을 볼 수 있다. C6, C7에 작은 돌출, C4, C5에 약간의 부풀어 오름과 T3, T4에 작은 중간 정도의 추간판 돌출, 그리고 갑상선에 다수의 낭종. 이러한 이유로 갑상선 초음파 검사를 실시하였고 갑상선에 단순한 덩어리나 낭종 등 다수의 혹들이 발견되었다. 오른쪽에 가장 큰 덩어리는 2.1×1.1×1.5cm 크기이고, 이는 혈관의 순환을 증가시킨다.
왼쪽에 있는 덩어리는 1.3×0.8×1.2 크기이고 이 또한 순환을 증가시킨다. 왼쪽협부의 복합 낭종 덩어리(크기)는 1.2×1.2×0.8. 환자는 좀 더 자세한 검진을 위해 방문하였다. 그녀의 갑상선 자극 호르몬 분비는 정상이다. 그녀는 극심한 피로를 호소하였으나 우울감이나 심각한 건망증은 없다고 했다. 그녀의 모발이 가늘어지기는 했으나 눈썹의 모발은 가늘어지지 않았다고 했다. 지난 몇 년간 체중이 약 22파운드 증가하였다. 그녀는 따뜻한 날씨를 선호하고, 종종 방도 따뜻한 것을 더 좋아한다. 손톱이 잘 부러진다고 호소한다. 변비도 있다. 환자는 20년 전 월경 과다로 인해 자궁 적출 수술을 받았다. 환자는 음식을 삼키는 데는 문제가 없으나 약을 삼키는 데 어려움을 겪는다고 했다. 복용하는 약으로는 필요에 따라 사용하는 이부프로펜 한 가지뿐이다.

과거 병력과 수술 경력:
당뇨병, 고혈압, 소화성 궤양, 담석증, 신석증, 류머티스성 열, 결핵, 심장마비 혹은 간질 증세 없음.

기관별 검진:
머리: 앞서 말한 바와 같이 두통 증세. 특별히 머리 뒤쪽에서부터 오른쪽 어깨까지 통증이 있고, 이 통증과 가끔씩 느끼는 손의 마비 증세는 관련이 있다. 별다른 증세 없음. **눈, 코, 목:** 이명이나 연하곤란 증세 없음. **폐:** 종종 숨가쁨. **심근계:** 가슴 통증이나 불규칙한 심장 박동은 없다고 함. **소화기계:** 자주 속이 쓰림. **생식기계:** 특이할 만한 사항은 없으나 폐경.
근골격계: 가끔씩 관절에 통증이 있고 걷기 시작할 때 통증을 느낀다. **신경계:** 가끔씩 발가락에 저린 느낌.

가족력:
할머니가 당뇨병, 어머니가 골다공증 앓음.
경력:
환자는 제조업 회사에서 사무직 일을 하고, 그녀의 남편은 신문사 편집자로 일한다.

다음 페이지 2에서 계속

Chart Note ② Endocrinology 내분비학과 영문본

ENDOCRINOLOGY

REFERRING PHYSICIAN: Dr. Richard Hann

CHIEF COMPLAINT: Thyroid nodule

HISTORY OF PRESENT ILLNESS:

Patricia is a 53 year old female, who as had significant head discomfort and pain. Had MRI of head that showed degenerative changes and disc protrusion at C5, C6 with flattening of the cord. Small protrusion at C6, C7. Mild budging C4, C5 and small medium disc protrusion T3, T4 and multiple cysts in thyroid gland. Because of this, a thyroid ultrasound was obtained that showed multinodular thyroid gland with non specific masses or cysts throughout the gland The largest mass in right was noted to be 2.1×1.1×1.5 cm with increased vascular flow.

Another mass on left was measured at 1.3×0.8×1.2, also increased flow. Complex cystic mass in left isthmus measuring 1.2×1.2×0.8. Patient was referred here for further evaluation. She had one TSH in normal range. She does complain of some fatigue, denies depression, denies significant forgetfulness. Has noticed her hair thinner, denies eyebrow thinning. Gaining apx 22Ibs in past few years. She prefers warm weather, occasionally prefers rooms warmer, Does complain of brittle nails. Does have constipation. She had hysterectomy for menorrhagia around 20 years ago. She has no difficulty swallowing food, but doe shave some trouble swallowing pills. Meds include only ibuprofen p.r.n.

PAST MEDICAL & SURGICAL HISTORY:

Negative for diabetes, hypertension, peptic ulcer disease, gall stones, kidney stones, rheumatic fever, tuberculosis, MI or seizures.

REVIEW OR SYSTEMS:

HEAD: Has headaches as noted. Specifically in back of head radiating down into right shoulders, associated with some numbness in her hands which seems to come and go. **EYES:** No complains. **ENT:** Denies tinnitus or significant dysphagia. **PUL:** Occasional shortness of breath. **CVS:** Denies chest pain or heart irregularities. **GI:** Complains of frequent heartburn. **GU:** No complaints except as noted. Has amenorrhea. **M/S:** Complains of occasional joint pain and foot pain when starting to walk. **NEURO:** Occasional tingling in toes.

FAMILY HISTORY:

Positive for diabetes in grandparents, osteoporosis in mother.

SOCIAL HISTORY:

Patient worked as office worker for Manufacturing Company. her husband works as a Newspaper Editor.

continued page 2

Chart Note ② Endocrinology 내분비학과 한글본

내분비학과

건강검진: 건강한 백인 여성으로 급성통증 소견은 없음.

혈압: 100/62. **맥박:** 60 정도. 규칙적 **체중:** 180파운드. **키:** 5.7인치. **눈:** 눈동자는 빛과 수정체 조절에 동일하게 반응한다. **이비인후:** 특이사항 없음. **목:** 갑상선은 촉진할 수 있고, 결절성. **호흡기:** 폐는 앞, 뒷부분에서 모두 기식을 동반하지 않고 호흡이 깨끗하다. **순환기:** 정상적 동리듬, 심잡음, 마찰음, 심장의 무질서한 박동 없음, 경동맥에 이상음 없음.

소화기: 특이사항 없음. 대장음 정상. **근골격계:** 부종, 곤봉증, 청색증 없음.

신경계: 건강. 고유 감각, 진동과 가벼운 접촉 모두 정상반응.

평가:

1. 다결절성 갑상샘종 두드러진 결절이 나타나서 조직을 떼어 냈고, 검사를 실시하도록 조처를 취할 것이다.
2. 하시모토병은 제외시켜야 함(하시모토병이 아닌지 판정해야 함). 조직검사 결과 음성이고 갑상선 항체가 양성이면 갑상선 호르몬치료를 시작할 수 있겠다. 만약 갑상선 항체가 음성이더라도 갑상선 호르몬의 징후일 수 있다. 환자의 갑상선 호르몬 치료를 방해하고 억제시킬 수 있는 다결절성 갑상샘종 형성의 병리생리학적 고찰을 했다.
3. 경추에 심각한 노화에 따른 변화
4. 두통 증세

계획: 갑상선 기능, 항핵항체, 비타민 B-12, 갑상선 항체, 코티졸(부신 피질 호르몬) 생화학 검사 실시. 실험적으로 6~8주 후에 환자 재검진. 만약 초음파 검사가 진단을 못하거나 양성일 경우, 그리고 다른 비정상 소견이 없을 경우: 갑상선 호르몬 치료가 적용될 수 있다.

Chart Note ② Endocrinology 내분비학과 영문본

ENDOCRINOLOGY

PHYSICAL EXAM: Shows a pleasant, white female in no acute distress.
BP: 100/62 **pulse:** 60 regular. **WT:** 180Lb **HT:** 5′7″. **EYES:** Pupils equally react to light and accommodation. **ENT:** Unremarkable. **NECK:** Thyroid is palpable and nodular. **PUL:** Lungs are clear to A & P. **CVS:** Regular sinus rhythm without murmurs, rubs or gallops. No carotid bruits.
ABD: Unremarkable. Bowel sounds are normal. **M/S:** No edema, clubbing or cyanosis.
NEURO: Intact. Proprioception, vibration and light touch are intact.

ASSESSMENT:

1. Multinodular goiter. There does appear to be dominant nodule so this should be biopsied. Will arrange for that to be done.
2. Rule out Hashimoto's disease. If biopsy is negative and if her thyroid antibodies are positive, one could make a case for starting thyroid hormone. Even if thyroid antibodies are negative, thyroid hormone might be indicated. We've reviewed with her the presumed pathphysiology of multinodular goiter formation, which may be interrupted and suppressed with thyroid hormone treatment.
3. Significant degenerative changes in cervical spine
4. Headaches as noted

PLAN: Thyroid functions, and repeat ANA, B-12, thyroid antibodies, cortisol, chemistries. Empirically see patient back in 6-8 weeks, If ultrasound is non diagnostic or benign and there is no other abnormalities: then thyroid hormone treatment would still be indicated.

단어 정리

☐ endocrinology	☐ 내분비학과
☐ referring physician	☐ 추천해 준 의사
☐ chief complaint	☐ 주증상
☐ history of present illness	☐ 현 병력
☐ degenerative	☐ 퇴행성의
☐ budge	☐ (조금) 움직이다
☐ protrusion	☐ 돌출, 융기
☐ cyst	☐ 낭포, 낭종
☐ gland	☐ 〈해부〉 선, 샘
☐ vascular	☐ 〈생물〉 도관(혈관)의(이 있는)
☐ isthmus	☐ 〈해부·동물〉 협부
☐ nodule	☐ 〈해부〉 소결절, 작은 혹(마디)
☐ fatigue	☐ (심신의) 피로, 피곤
☐ depression	☐ 우울증
☐ brittle nails	☐ 쉽게 부서지는 손톱
☐ hysterectomy	☐ 자궁 절제(술)
☐ menorrhagia	☐ 〈생리〉 (정상적인) 월경, 〈병리〉 월경과다(증)
☐ tuberculosis	☐ 결핵
☐ diabetes	☐ 당뇨
☐ hypertension	☐ 고혈압
☐ ulcer	☐ 궤양
☐ gall stone	☐ 담석
☐ kidney stone	☐ 신석
☐ rheumatic fever	☐ 류머티스성 열
☐ seizure	☐ 발작
☐ dysphagia	☐ 〈병리〉 부전실어증
☐ amenorrhea	☐ 〈병리〉 무월경, 월경폐지
☐ osteoporosis	☐ 골다공증
☐ A & P(Anterior and Posterior): anterior	☐ 앞면의
☐ P & A(Anterior and Posterior): posterior	☐ 뒷면의
☐ murmurs	☐ 심잡음

☐ rubs	☐ 마찰(음)
☐ gallops	☐ 분마율, 심장의 무질서한 율동
☐ carotid	☐ 목동맥-, 경동맥-
☐ bruits	☐ (청진기로 들을 수 있는) 이상음
☐ bowel sound	☐ 대장음
☐ Proprioception	☐ 고유 감각
☐ vibration	☐ 진동
☐ pathphysiology	☐ 병태생리학, 병리생리학
☐ multinodular	☐ 다결절성
☐ goiter	☐ 갑상샘종
☐ formation	☐ 형성

Chart Note ③ Urology 비뇨기과 한글본

비뇨기과

9월 9일 (환자 이름)

주증상: 1) 전립선 매년 정기검진. 2) 느린 배뇨. 3) 야뇨증: 매 2시간 내지 4시간마다.
환자는 8~9년 전 경요도 절제술 이후 계속적으로 소변 줄기가 약해졌다. 그는 방광경 검사를 하였고 요도는 열려 있다. 그는 특별히 의학적 치료 방법으로 선택할 수 있는 방법들이 있는지 알고 싶어 한다. 그는 열, 오한, 배뇨장애, 혈뇨증세가 없다.

기관별 검사
약: 아스피린과 다이아자이드
신체검사: 그는 외견상 건강하고 밝은 남성이다.
목에는 결절이나 덩어리 없음, 호흡도 깨끗하다. 복부는 덩어리나 압통은 없으나 약간 볼록하다. 간 지라비대증 없음. 서혜부에 탈장 없음. (남성)성기는 정상이고 포경수술이 되어 있다. 고환은 하강되어 있다. 항문은 매우 협착하고 1+ 전립선 비대이며 치질 없음, 긴장도 좋음.
신경의학적인 정신치료 3회. 소변 검사결과 이상 없음.

검토: 나(의사)는 카두라(약)를 하루 1밀리그램씩 일주일간, 2주째는 2밀리그램씩, 그 이후는 4밀리그램씩 복용해 볼 것을 제안하였다. 그는 변화되었는지 보기 위해 한 달 후 재방문할 것이다. 그의 소변 검사는 깨끗하다. 그는 약국에서 일하는 딸이 있어서 이 증세에 대해 같이 관찰을 할 것이다.

의사 서명

다음 페이지 2에서 계속

Chart Note ③ Urology 비뇨기과 영문본

Urology

09/09/_____ JOHNNY DOE

CHIEF COMPLAINT: 1) Yearly prostate check. 2) Slow urination. 3) Nocturia q. two to four hours. Patient has had persistent slowing of his stream since we did the TUR nearly eight to nine years ago. He had a cystoscopy. He asked for options, especially medical treatment. He has no fevers, chills, dysuria, or hematuria.

REVIEW OF SYSTEMS:
MEDICATIONS: Aspirin and Dyazide.
PHYSICAL EXAMINATION: He is a healthy appearing, very bright male.
Neck without nodes or mass. Respirations are clear. Abdomen is slightly protuberant without masses or tenderness. No hepatosplenomegaly. Inguinal without hernia. Penis is normal and circumcised. Testis are descended. Rectal is a really small, 1+, benign prostate without hemorrhoids and good tone. Neuropsych is oriented times three. His urinalysis is negative.

DISCUSSION: I offered a trial of Cardura beginning with 1 mg daily for a week, progressing to 2 mg in two weeks, and then to 4 mg.
He will return in a month to see if we have made any progress. His urinalysis is clear. He does have a daughter in pharmacy who will monitor these symptoms as well.

__________, M.D./ht: ____

continued page 2

Chart Note ③ Urology 비뇨기과 한글본

비뇨기과

존은 나의 전화에 응답하였다. 나는 그의 L1 압박 골절에 대해 의논하였다. 환자는 지난 11월 사다리에서 떨어져 허리를 다친 이후 생긴 통증이 남아 있기는 하나 허리는 괜찮다고 말했다. 나는 T11에 대하여 말하였다. 환자는 잘 지내고 있고 다음 재진에 오고 싶지 않다고 한다. 그는 허리의 압박 골절에 대해서 그리고 전립선암에 대해 잘 이해하고 있다. 그는 약속한 대로 다시 방문할 것이다.

의사 서명

존은 전립선 특이항원의 증가에 대해 검사 받기 위해 병원에 재방문하였다. 그는 지난 가을 이후로 출혈은 더 이상 없었다. 소변 줄기가 건강하게 배뇨를 하고 있다. 그는 소변이 급하거나, 빈뇨, 배뇨장애, 혈뇨 또는 다른 문제는 없다.

신체검사: 전립선은 +2에서 +3, 비대칭, 오른쪽이 왼쪽보다 훨씬 더 비대. 그리고 조금 더 단단함. 소변검사 정상.

환자와 병에 대한 소견을 나누었다. 나는 전립선 특이항원과 전립선암과의 관계에 대해 말했다. 나는 그의 과거 병리에 대해 말했다. 환자는 보존적인 치료를 원한다. 그는 그의 전립선 특이항원 결과를 알기 위해 전화를 할 것이다. 그는 다른 문제가 있거나 출혈, 혹은 그 외 고통이 있을 때 나에게 전화를 할 것이다.

의사 서명

환자는 오늘 전립선 재검진을 위해 병원에 방문하였다. 그는 그의 양성 전립선 비대가 예전처럼 괴롭히지 않는다고 한다. 그는 다른 증세는 없다고 한다. 소변검사는 정상이다.

신체검사: 전립선은 +2 양성, 전립선 특이항원은 아직 미결정 상태이다. 환자는 결과를 알기 위해 전화를 할 것이다. 환자는 1년 후에 재방문할 것이다.

의사 서명

Chart Note ③ Urology 비뇨기과 영문본

Urology

10/__/____ JOHN DOE

John returned my call today. I talked to him about his compression fracture of L1. The patient says that his back feels fine except for a little residual pain he has had since he fell off his ladder and hurt his back in November. I talked to him about T11. The patient says he is doing well and does not desire to see me in follow-up. He understands about the compression fractures of his back and about his advancing prostate cancer. He will see me again as scheduled.

__________, M.D./ht:slh

12/__/____ JOHN DOE

John returns to the clinic today for further evaluation of his elevated PSA. He has had no further bleeding since last fall. He is voiding well with a good force of stream. He has no urgency, frequency, dysuria, hematuria, or other problems.

PHYSICAL EXAMINATION: Prostate is +2 to +3, asymmetrical, right much greater than left, slightly firmer. Urinalysis is negative.

Discussed my findings with the patient. I talked to him about the association of PSA with prostate cancer. I talked to him about his previous pathology. The patient desires conservative follow-up. He will call for the results of his PSA. He will call me with further problems, bleeding, or other difficulties.

__________, M.D./ht:slh

12/__/_____ JOHN DOE #00-00-00-6

The patient returns to the clinic today for a prostate recheck. His benign prostatic hypertrophy is not bothering him anymore than it was. He denies any other symptoms. Urinalysis is negative.

PHYSICAL EXAMINATION: Prostate is +2, benign. PSA is pending. The patient will call for the results. He will return to the clinic in one year.

__________, M.D./ht:slh

Chart Note ③ Urology 비뇨기과 한글본

비뇨기과

04/__/_____ (환자 이름)

존은 질문이나 문제 없이 병원을 방문하였다.
그는 좋아 보였다. 그는 어려움 없이 배뇨를 하고 있다.
신체검사: 전립선 +2에서 +3 양성 소변검사는 정상.
전립선 특이항원 아직 미결정.
앞으로의 치료에 대해 의견 교환했다. 그는 1년 후 재방문할 것이다. 그리고 전립선 특이항원에 대해 전화를 할 것이다.

의사 서명__________

09/__/_____ (환자 이름)

존은 미세혈뇨에 대해 더 검진하기 위해 내원하였다. 경정맥성 신우 촬영술(Intrabenous Pyelography)은 돌출한 전립선을 보이는 것 외에는 정상이다. 경정맥성 신우 촬영술은 정상 요도의 세엽 과다 증식과 다소의 방광 경부 충혈을 보여 준다. 방광 경부의 가벼운 출혈이 방광경 검사를 어렵게 만들었다.
뚜렷한 병변은 없다. 환자와 소견에 대해 의논하였다. 레바퀸(약) 250밀리, 하루 4번 구강으로 복용하도록 하고 약의 부작용에 대해 알려 주었다.
그는 알고 있는 바에 의하면 알레르기 반응은 없다. 나는 6주 후에 방광경 재검사를 위해 환자를 다시 볼 것이다. 만약 그가 질문이나 문제가 있으면 그 전에라도 전화를 할 것이다.

의사 서명__________

03/__/____ (환자 이름)

존은 방사선 치료 후의 상태를 검진하러 내원하였다. 그는 혈뇨증이나 소변이 급하거나, 빈뇨, 배뇨장애 설사 혹은 매슥거림이나 구토 증세는 없다. 그는 건강하다.
신체검사: 그는 심한 통증이 없는 건강한 사람이다. 소변 검사는 정상이다. 전립선 특이항원(Prostate Specific Antigen) 검사를 실시했고 아직 미결정 상태이다. 환자가 결과를 알기 위해 전화할 것이다. 그는 6개월 내에 다시 내원할 것이다.

의사 서명__________

Chart Note ③ Urology 비뇨기과 영문본

Urology

04/__/_____ JOHN DOE #00-00-0-3

John returns to the clinic today without questions or problems.
He is doing well. He is voiding well without difficulty.
PHYSICAL EXAMINATION: Prostate is +2 to +3, benign. Urinalysis is negative.
PSA is pending.
Discussed follow-up with the patient. He will return to the clinic in one year. He will call for the results of his PSA.

__________, M.D./ht:slh

09/__/_____ JOHN DOE #0-00-00-8

John returns to the clinic today for further evaluation of a trace amount of microscopic hematuria.
IVP is normal showing prominent prostate.
Cystoscopy reveals normal urethra with obvious trilobar hyperplasia and a somewhat irritated bladder neck. Mild bleeding from the bladder neck made cystoscopy difficult. There were no obvious lesions.
Discussed findings with the patient. Levaquin 250 mg p.o. q. day for four days was given. A prescription for a week after that was given and complications of the medication was discussed. He has no known medical ALLERGIES.
I will see again in six weeks for a repeat cystoscopy. He will call sooner with questions or problems.

__________, M.D./ht:slh

03/__/____ JOHN L. DOE #00-00-00-6

John returns to the clinic today status post radiation. He is having no hematuria, urgency, frequency, dysuria, diarrhea, or immediate nausea and vomiting. He feels well.
PHYSICAL EXAMINATION: He is a healthy individual in no acute distress.
Urinalysis is negative. PSA is drawn and pending. The patient will call for the results.
He will return to the clinic in six months.

__________, M.D./ht:slh

단어 정리

□ Trans-Urethral Resection	□ 경요도 절제술
□ *Cystoscopy	□ *방광경 검사
□ dyura	□ 〈병리〉 배뇨(排尿) 장애[곤란]
□ hematuria [hmti, hm-]	□ 〈병리〉 혈뇨증(血尿症)
□ protuberant [proutbrnt, pr-/prtj-]	□ 돌출[돌기]한, 불룩한, 융기한
□ hepatosplenomegaly	□ 간지라비대, 간비장비대
□ inguinal [gwnl]	□ 〈해부·병리〉 서혜(鼠蹊)(부)의
□ circumcised [skmsizd]	□ 할례받은, 포경수술을 받은
□ descended testis	□ 하강 고환
□ prostate	□ 〈해부〉 전립선(前立腺)의, 전립선- (gland); 〈구어〉 전립선 이상
□ Benign Prostatic Hyperplasia(BPH)	□ 전립선 비대
□ hemorrhoids	□ 〈복수취급〉〈병리〉 치질, 치핵
□ neuropsychiatry	□ 신경정신과학, 신경정신의학
□ compression fracture	□ 압박골절
□ residual	□ 남겨진, 나머지의, 잔류의
□ PSA: [Prostate(Prostatic)-Specific Antigen]	□ 전립선 특이항원
□ urine frequency	□ 빈뇨
□ dysuria	□ 배뇨장애
□ asymmetrical	□ 비대칭의
□ prostate cancer	□ 전립선암
□ pathology	□ 1. 병리학 2. 병리, 병상(病狀) 3. 비정상
□ hypertrophy	□ 비대

* 참고
방광경 검사란 방광을 비롯해 방광으로부터 소변을 배출하는 관인 요도 내부를 관찰하기 위한 처치입니다. 방광경 기계는 관상형 기구로 렌즈, 카메라, 한쪽 면에 광원과 다른 쪽의 접안경을 가지고 있습니다. 이 기구를 이용하여 요도와 방광 내부를 관찰할 수 있습니다.

Chart Note ④ Orthopedics 정형외과 한글본

정형외과

페더럴웨이 정형외과
의사, Mike Zhivago
워싱턴주 시애틀
(206) 555-2222

환자: Remond Kandell
날짜: 2003년 6월 20일
보낸 의사: 의사, Jekyll

주요 증상: 오른쪽 무릎 통증

통증기간: 6개월간 통증 심화와 불안정성

임상치료과정: 인대 재건 수술, 1962년 6개월 전까지는 아무 문제 없었음. 최근 엑스레이는 골극(군뼈)과 3~4단계의 골관절염과 함께 관절 간 어느 정도의 협착 소견을 보여 준다.

신체검사: 오른쪽 무릎 검진결과 내측 관절선 압통을 보여 준다. 환자는 관찰 결과 심각한 내반 변형을 보여 준다.

기능의 제한성: 환자는 더 이상 오락적인 산책이나 운동을 할 수 없게 되었다.

치료 내력: 진통효과 없이 신비스크(골관절염에 쓰이는 약) 주사 투여. 셀리브렉스(골관절염에 먹는 약)로 다소의 진통 효과를 보았다.

예후: 환자는 현재 수술은 피하고 싶어 한다. 결국에는 대퇴골(무릎) 교체 수술을 해야 할 것이다.

권고사항: 셀리브렉스 계속 복용과 개인에 맞추어 제작되는 무릎 보조 장치를 추천한다. 이 보조 장치는 심각한 내반 변형을 위해 필요하게 될 것이다.

의사, Zhivago

2005년 3월 21일

Chart Note ④ Orthopedics 정형외과 영문본

Orthopedics

Federal Way Orthopedics
Mike Zhivago, M.D.
1234 56thSt.
Seattle, WA 78910
(206) 555-2222

Patient: Remond Kandell
Date: June 20, 2003
Referring Physician: Dr. Jekyll

Chief Complaint: Right knee pain

Duration: Increased pain and instability for six months

Clinical Course: Ligament reconstruction surgery, 1962 with no problems until 6 months ago. Recent x-ray shows moderate joint space narrowing with osteophytes, indicative of grade 3-4 osteoarthritis.

Physical Exam: Right knee exam demonstrated significant medial joint line tenderness. On observation, Patient has severe varus deformity right knee.

Functional limitations: Patient no longer able to participate in recreational walks or exercise.

Previous Treatments: Synvisc injections with no pain relief. Celebrex gave some pain relief.

Prognosis: Patient would like to avoid surgery for now. Will eventually need total knee replacement.

Recommend: Continue Celebrex and refer patient for GII Custom Fabricated Unloader knee brace. Custom brace will be needed because of severity of varus deformity.

Dr. Zhivago

March 21, 2005

단어 정리

□ instability	□ 〈물리〉 불안정성[상태]
□ ligament reconstruction surgery	□ 인대복원수술
□ osteophytes	□ 골 증식체, 뼈(골)돌기(골의 병적 증식물)
□ osteoarthritis	□ 골관절염
□ medial	□ 안쪽의, 내측의
□ varus deformity	□ (달리 분류되지 않은) 내반 변형
□ severity	□ 중대성, 심각성

Chart Note ⑤ Family Medicine 가정의학과 한글본

이름: 릴리 매 젠킨스
생년월일: 1922년 3월 7일
(진료)날짜: 2011년 1월 11일:

가정의학과
닥터 고든 벤더

환자 내력
주요증세: 항문 출혈, 하루 경과
현 병력: 어젯 밤, 선홍색의 피가 섞인 변을 보았다. 오늘 아침, 다시 대변을 보았고, 거의 선홍색의 피였다. 그녀는 50년 전에 담낭 질환을 앓은 내력이 있다. 그녀는 담낭 제거에 대해 거절하였고 그 이후 저지방식을 해오고 있다. 그녀의 딸은, 환자에게 여러 번의 담낭 질환의 발병이 있었고, 이것은 며칠간 지속되며, 오른쪽 상복부에 심한 통증을 느꼈다고 했다.
그녀는 담낭 질환과는 다르게 때때로, 오른쪽 하복부에 간헐적인 통증을 느꼈다고 한다.

과거 병력
수술: 1997년 그녀는 왼쪽 안구적출술을 받았다. 그녀는 2005년 오른쪽 눈에 녹내장 수술을 받았다.
진료: 1986년 오른팔 콜레스골절. 척추에 심각한 관절염.
복용약: 환자는 현재 하루에 에비스타 60 밀리그램, 매일 아침 플라빅스 75 밀리그램, 인도신 한 알씩 하루 3회. 그녀는 통증이 있을 때는, 필요시 버파린을 복용한다. 그녀는 지난 5년간 니트로글리세린을 일주일에 2~3알씩 계속 복용해 왔다.

가족력: 환자의 부모 모두 80세 이상까지 사셨다. 그녀는 6명의 자녀를 두었다. 자녀 하나는 3세에 자동차 사고로 입은 부상으로 인해 사망했다. 자녀 하나는 유방암으로 56세에 사망했다. 그 외에 다른 특이할 만한 사항은 없다.

기능별 진단:
머리, 눈, 귀 코, 목: 오른쪽 청력 상실, 왼쪽 청력 감소. 왼쪽눈 인공안구, 오른쪽눈 약간의 시력만 남아 있어서 물체가 정중앙에 있을 때만 볼 수 있음. 환자는 몇 년째 무치아 상태였다.
가슴: 비흡연자
심혈관: 환자는 지난 5년간 협심증이 있었고, 지난 3년간 비정상 심장도를 나타냈다. 그녀는 항상 감기를 앓고 있으며 체온을 유지하려고 늘 몸을 웅크리고 있다.
위장: 배변 정상. 현 병력 참조.
비뇨생식기: 그녀는 지난해 신부전이 발병했음에도 불구하고 신장 방광이나 신장 감염은 없다.
신경근육계: 환자는 척추에 다소 무기력하게 만드는 욱신욱신하고 심각한 통증을 느끼고 있으나 버파린을 복용하면서 그럭저럭 견디고 있다.

Chart Note ⑤ Family Medicine 가정의학과 영문본

Name: Lily Mae Jenkins
DOB: March, 7th 1922
date: Jan. 11th 2011

Family Medicine
Gordon Bender, MD

CHIEF COMPLAINT: Rectal Bleeding, X one day

PRESENT ILLNESS:

Last night, she had a bowel movement that had some bright-red blood mixed in with it. This morning, she had another bowel movement, and it consisted mostly of bright-red blood. She has a history of gallbladder disease, dating back over 50 years. She refused to have her gallbladder taken out but has been on a low-fat diet ever since that time. Her daughter describes numerous gallbladder attacks, lasting for several days, consisting of severe, right-upper quadrant pain. She has had occasional, intermittent right lower quadrant pain that does not seem similar to the gallbladder attacks.

PAST HISTORY

Operations: In 1997, she had enucleation of the left eye. She had surgery in 2005 for glaucoma in the right eye. **Medical:** 1986, Colles' fracture, right wrist. 1990s, severe arthritis of her spine. **Medications:** Patient is presently taking Evista 60mg per day, Plavix 75mg every morning, Indocin 1 tablet t.i.d. She takes Bufferin p.r.n. for pain. She takes nitroglycerin 2-3 tablets per week for chest pain and has done so for 5 years.

FAMILY: Both of her parents lived until their 80s. She had 6 children: 1 died at age 3. The result of injuries sustained in and automobile accident: 1 died at age 56 of carcinoma of the breast. Otherwise, the family history is unremarkable. There are 4 children who are alive and well.

FUNCTIONAL INQUIRY:

HEENT: Hearing in her right ear is absent. Hearing in her left ear is decreased. There is an artificial eye in the left, and there is only slight vision in her right eye if one comes exactly in the middle of her visual field. Patient has been edentulous for several years.

CHEST: Nonsmoker

CV: Patient has had angina for over 5 years and abnormal cardiograms for the last 3 years. She is cold all of the time and is constantly bundling herself up in and effort to keep warm.

GI: Her bowel movements have been normal. See Present illness.

GU: She has no history of any bladder or kidney infections, despite the fact that she had a history of kidney failure last ear.

NM: Patient has shooing, severe pains up her spine that are relatively incapacitating, but she manages to keep going by just taking Bufferin.

Chart Note ⑥ PHYSICAL EXAMINATION 신체검사 한글본

이름: 릴리 매 젠킨스
생년월일: 1922년 3월 7일
(진료)날짜: 2011년 1월 11일

신체검사

일반: 이는 90세의 여성으로 특정 질병은 없고 청력이 약하지만 질문에는 답할 수 있다.

목: 경동맥 잡음 없음. 경정맥 팽만 없음. 갑상선 촉지할 수 있고, 이상 없음. 목의 운동범위가 약간 제한적이다.

가슴: 촉진이나 청진 결과 깨끗함.
심장: 심첨박동 감지할 수 없음. 왼쪽 늑연골부의 연골에 다소의 압통이 있음. 타진에는 심장 크기의 확대 없음. 분명치 않은 심장음이 있음. 3번째, 4번째 심음 없음. 바로 누운 자세에서 심잡음 없음.
유방: 촉진 혹(덩어리) 소견이 없음.

복부: 부드러움. 복벽에 노인성 각화증 소견 없음. 오른쪽 하복부 깊이 촉진하면 막창자 주위에 광범위한 압통을 보였다. 그 외에 복부에서 압통이나 비정상적인 장음이 발견된 바 없었다. 장음은 정상 범위에 속한다.

골반: 실시하지 않음.

직장: 전체 S상 결장경 검사결과 25센티미터 지점의 S상 결장에서 확실한 출혈지점은 확인되지 않았지만 신선혈이 발견되었다.

사지: 등은 사실상 움직일 수 없음. 고관절 운동성 통증 없고 정상 범위. 오로지 +1 오른쪽 발등 맥박만 있고 말단부 맥박은 나타나지 않음. 양쪽 발이 현저한 냉기가 있음.

중추 신경계: 환자의 근력은 정상 범위. 반사작용 정상 범위. 수족 운동위 협조기능 검사 실시하지 않음. 파킨슨병으로 인한 불수의 떨림이 있다.

진단: 1. 급성 위장출혈, 병인 아직 진단하지 못함
2. 만성 담낭염
3. 심각한 척추 골관절염
4. 협심증이 동반된 동맥경화심장병

Chart Note ⑥ PHYSICAL EXAMINATION 신체검사 영문본

Name: Lily Mae Jenkins
DOB: March, 7th 1922
date: Jan. 11th 2011

PHYSICAL EXAMINATION

GENERAL: This is a 90-year-old woman in no obvious distress, who is hard of hearing but can answer questions.

NECK: There are no carotid bruits. No jugular venous distention. Thyroid is palpable and unremarkable. Range of motion of the neck is generally slightly restricted.

CHEST: Clear on percussion and auscultation.
HEART: The apical beat is not palpable. There is some tenderness over the costochondral cartilages on the left side. Heart size is not enlarged to percussion. There is muffled heart sound. There is no 3rd or 4th heart sound. There are no murmurs heard in the supine position.
BREAST: Palpable. and there are no masses noted.

ABDOMEN: Soft. There are marked senile keratoses over the abdominal wall. There is some diffuse tenderness on deep palpation over the cecum in the right lover quadrant. There is no other tenderness noted or abnormal bowel sounds noted in the abdomen. Bowel sounds are within normal limits.

PELVIC: Not done.

RECTAL: Full sigmoidoscopic examination to 25 cm revealed fresh blood in the sigmoid area with no obvious bleeding source noted.

EXTREMITIES: There is essentially no motion in the back. Range of motion of the hips is within normal limits and painless. There is only a + 1 dorsalis pedis on the right: otherwise, there are no peripheral pulses present. There is marked coldness of both feet.

CENTRAL NERVOUS SYSTEM: The patient's strength is within normal limits. The reflexes are within normal limits. Coordination is not tested. There is and involuntary shaking, consistent with the diagnosis of old Parkinson disease.

IMPRESSION:
1. Acute gastrointestinal hemorrhage, etiology not yet diagnosed
2. Chronic cholecystitis
3. Severe osteoarthritis of spine
4. Arteriosclerotic heart disease with angina pectoris

단어 정리

☐ enucleation	☐ 1. 안구적출(술) 2. 적출 3. 핵제거
☐ Colles' fracture	☐ 콜레스골절
☐ edentulous	☐ 무치아
☐ cardiogram	☐ 심장도
☐ GI(Gastro-Intestinal)	☐ 위장의
☐ GU(Genito-Urinary)	☐ 비뇨생식기의
☐ NM(Neuro-Muscular)	☐ 신경 근육계의
☐ kidney failure	☐ 신부전(不全)
☐ incapacitating	☐ 무능력하게 된
☐ central nervous system	☐ 중추신경계통, 중추신경계
☐ carotid bruit	☐ 목동맥잡음, 경동맥잡음
☐ jugular venous	☐ 목정맥, 경정맥
☐ distention	☐ 팽만, 팽창
☐ palpable	☐ 촉지할 수 있는
☐ range of motion	☐ 운동범위
☐ apical impulse	☐ 심장꼭대기박동, 심첨박동
☐ percussion	☐ 타진
☐ costochondral	☐ 갈비연골-, 늑연골
☐ cartilages	☐ 연골
☐ supine position	☐ 바로누운자세, 앙와위
☐ murmurs	☐ 심장잡음
☐ senile keratosis	☐ 노인성 각화증(老人性 角化症)
☐ abdominal wall	☐ 배벽, 복벽
☐ diffuse	☐ 광범위-, 확산-, 미만-
☐ tenderness	☐ 압통, 누름통증
☐ cecum	☐ 막창자, 맹장
☐ normal limit	☐ 정상한계
☐ dorsalis	☐ 등쪽 부분, 배측부
☐ dorsalis pedis(artery)	☐ 발등동맥
☐ peripheral	☐ 말초방향으로, 말초의
☐ coordination test	☐ 수족협조기능검사(手足協調機能檢査), (근육 운동의) 공동 작업

☐ involuntary	☐ 불수의(不隨意)의, 무의식의
☐ gastrointestinal hemorrhage	☐ 위창자출혈, 위장출혈
☐ etiology	☐ 병인론, 병인(병의 원인)
☐ cholecystitis	☐ 쓸개염, 담낭염
☐ osteoarthritis	☐ 골관절염
☐ arteriosclerotic heart disease	☐ 동맥경화심장병

Chart Note ⑦ PATIENT'S RECORDS 환자 진료기록 한글본 【1】

환자 진료기록

이름: 레이몬드 파이퍼
생년월일: 2011년 3월 25일 4/26/2011

주관적 소견
어머니가 1개월 된 남자 아이를 데리고 왔다. 환자는 건강하다. 광선요법을 하고 있다. 환자는 목이 마르고, 노란색 건강한 대변을 보며, 우유(모유가 아닌)를 먹고 있다. 아이의 반응(각성도)은 정상이다. 다른 적절한 기관별 검진은 진단과 상관이 없다.

객관적 소견
열 없음. 편안한 상태. 지금 황달은 최소의 상태. 공막의 신생아황달 없음. 움직임 정상. 숫구멍(천문) 정상. 측두하악관절, 코, 입, 인두, 목, 심장, 폐, 복부, 간, 이자, 그리고 성기 모두 정상. 표피절개술(포경수술) 받았음. 사지 건강.

실시
병원 기록 받아서 검토
생체검진, 머리, 얼굴, 목, 가슴, 피부 등의 일반 검진 실시
예방주사 계획에 대해 검토
B형 간염 예방주사 (첫 회) 실시

계획
광선요법은 중단할 것이고, 2일 후에 다시 상승하는지 확실히 알기 위해 빌리루빈 수치를 검토한다. 환자는 일주일 후 다시 재진을 위해 방문할 것이다. 일상적 검진에 대해 논의하였다.

Chart Note ⑦ PATIENT'S RECORDS 환자 진료기록 영문본 【1】

PATIENT'S RECORDS

Name: Raymond Piper

DOB: March 25th, 2011 4/26/2011

SUBJECTIVE

The mother brought in this 1-month-old male. The patient is doing very well. They have been using the phototherapy blanket. He is thirsty, has good yellow stooling, and continues on formula. His alertness is normal. Other pertinent review of systems is noncontributory.

OBJECTIVE

Afebrile. Comfortable. Jaundice is only minimal at this time. No scleral icterus. Good activity level. Normal fontanel. TMs, nose, mouth, pharynx, neck, heart, lungs, abdomen, liver, spleen, and groins are normal. Circumcision. Good extremities.

ASSESSMENT

Hospital records were received and reviewed

Check vital signs, general appearance include head, face, neck, chest, skin

Discuss Vaccination Schedule

Hep N #1 injection given

PLAN

Will stop phototherapy and do a bilirubin level in a couple of days to make sure there is no rebound. The patient is to be seen in one week. Routine care was discussed.

단어 정리

☐ phototherapy	☐ 광선요법(光線療法)
☐ *formula	☐ *유아용혼합분유
☐ alertness	☐ 각성도, 민첩(敏捷)함
☐ noncontributory	☐ (의학) 진단에 도움이 안 되는
☐ afebrile	☐ 무열성(無熱性)의
☐ jaundice	☐ 황달
☐ scleral	☐ 공막(鞏膜)의
☐ icterus	☐ 신생아황달
☐ fontanel	☐ 숫구멍, 천문
☐ TMs+joint	☐ 측두하악관절
☐ pharynx	☐ 인두(혀뒷부분부터 후두와 식도 앞까지를 인두라 함)
☐ groins	☐ 성기(性器), 고환
☐ circumcision	☐ 윤절술, 포피 절개술, 포경수술
☐ bilirubin	☐ 빌리루빈(담즙의 주성분)

* 참고
formular fed: 분유를 먹이는 *breast fed 모유를 먹이는

Chart Note ⑦ PATIENT'S RECORDS 환자 진료기록 한글본 【2】

환자 진료기록

주요증상: 조는 왼쪽 무릎의 통증, 부종, 쇠약함을 갖고 병원을 처음 방문하였다. 그는 과거 이 부위에 상처는 없었으나 오른쪽 무릎 통증과 관절염을 갖고 있었다. 최근 보험 정책의 변경으로 인해 의사를 바꾸었다.

과거병력: 과거 병력 일반적으로 없음. **과거 수술경력:** 없음. **사회력:** 비흡연자. 그는 하루 4~6 캔의 맥주를 마신다. **가족력:** 아버지 퇴행성 디스크 질환 있고, 남자 형제는 척추후궁절제가 요구되는 탈출 추간판 증세를 갖고 있다.

복용약: 없음.

검진: 몸무게 304파운드. 첫 회 실시 혈압 134/104, 재실시 혈압 132/94.
왼쪽 무릎: 진찰결과 오른쪽에 비해 열이 나고 부어 있음이 관찰되었다.
신전은 180도, 굴곡은 90도 각도. 무릎 앞뒤 움직임 테스트 음성. 어플리 그라인드 테스트(무릎반달연골 검사), 그리고 파텔라 검사(무릎 슬개골 검사) 음성. 그는 압통과 슬개골과 슬개골상 인대 촉진 시 마찰음이 있다.
말초맥박: 말초맥박은 2+/4이고 다리오금, 뒤쪽 정강부위, 발등부분 대칭적.

엑스레이: 육안으로는 골절 혹은 이상 소견 없음.

검사: 공복이 아닌 경우의 혈당 120, 총 콜레스테롤 양 253, 요산 8.8

진단: 통풍성 관절염의 이차적인 증상으로 좌측 무릎통증과 부종.

계획:
데이프로(약) 600밀리그램 하루 2회 1주일 간. 알코올 섭취량 줄일 것.
1주일 후 재진. 호전되지 않으면 알로푸리놀(약) 복용을 시작할 것이다.

의사 조셉 블랙우드

Chart Note ⑦ PATIENT'S RECORDS 환자 진료기록 영문본 【2】

PATIENT'S RECORDS

CHIEF COMPLAINT: Joe is a new patient who present to the clinic with left knee pain, swelling, and weakness. He denies previous trauma to this area but has had right knee pain and arthritis in the past. Recently he changed physicians because of change in healthcare policies.

PAST MEDICAL HISTORY: Past history generally negative. **Past surgical history:** Negative. **Social history:** Nonsmoker. He does drink beer, 4 to 6 cans per day. **Family history:** Father has degenerative disk disease; brother had herniated disk, which required a laminectomy.

MEDICATIONS: None.

EXAMINATION: Weight 304 pounds. Initial BP 134/104; repeat 132/94.
LEFT KNEE: Exam showed the knee to be warm and swollen compared to right knee.
Extension is 180 degrees; flexion is 90degrees. Negative drawer. Apley grind, and patellar apprehension test. He has marked tenderness and crepitus in the patellar and suprapatellar ligament on palpation.
PERIPHERAL PULSES: They are 2+/4 and symmetrical in the popliteal, posterior tibial, and dorsalis pedis areas.

X-RAY: No gross evidence of fractures or abnormalities.

LABORATORY: Nonfasting glucose 120, total cholesterol 253, and uric acid 8.8

DIAGNOSIS:
Left knee pain and swelling secondary to gouty arthritis.

PLAN:
Daypro 600mg 2 daily for 1 week. Decrease alcohol consumption. Recheck in 1 week; if there is no improvement, he will start on allopurinol.

Joseph blackwood, MD

단어 정리

□ trauma	□ 외상(신체적 또는 정신적인 창상 또는 손상)
□ degenerative	□ 퇴행-, 변성-
□ herniated disc	□ 탈출추간판, 탈출척추원반
□ laminectomy	□ 척추후궁절제(술), 고리판절제(술)
□ extension	□ 1. 폄, 신전 2. 확장, 신장 3. 확대
□ flexion	□ 굽힘, 굴곡
□ apley grind test(or apley test)	□ 무릎반달연골 검사(used to evaluate individuals for problems in the meniscus of the knee)
□ knee draw test anterior/posterior	□ 무릎 전방/후방 움직임 검사
□ patellar apprehension test	□ 슬개골(불안감) 검사(evaluates for patellar subluxation or dislocation)
□ patellar	□ 슬개골
□ subluxation	□ 불완전탈구, 아탈구
□ dislocation	□ 탈구
□ crepitus	□ 비빔소리, 마찰음
□ suprapatellar	□ 슬개골상(膝蓋骨上)의
□ ligamenta	□ 인대(足側靭帶)
□ palpation	□ 촉진
□ peripheral pulse	□ 말초맥박(~脈搏)
□ popliteal	□ 다리오금-, 오금-
□ tibial	□ 정강뼈-, 정강-, 정강쪽-, 경골-
□ symmetrical	□ 대칭의, 대칭성의, 대측의
□ gross	□ 1. 큰 2. 맨눈-, 육안- 3. 거친
□ nonfasting	□ 공복이 아닌
□ gouty arthritis	□ 통풍(성) 관절염

* 참고
fasting blood sugar 공복혈당

환자 진료기록

산부인과
이름: 제인 ××××
생년월일: 1957년 4월 11일

제인은 심각한 얼굴 홍조(열감) 증세로 웰즈 의사에게 상담을 받았다. 환자는 52세이고, 백인이며 일년 전 마지막 월경이 있었고 그 이후로는 더 이상 출혈은 없었다. 그녀는 월경이 끊어지면서부터 얼굴 홍조 증세가 시작되었고 점점 더 악화되고 밤에 더욱 심하다고 한다. 그녀는 몹시 열이 나서 눕기가 꺼려진다고 말한다. 그녀는 한 시간에서 한 시간 반 정도 자고 나면 열감 때문에 잠이 깨고 일어나서 열을 식히기 위해 밖으로 나가기도 한다고 한다. 얼굴이 달아 오르는 것은 심한 발한(땀이 남)을 동반하고 밤에는 더욱 심하다. 그녀는 낮 동안에는 심하게 열이 날 때 밖으로 나가 식힐 수 있어 낮 시간 동안에 견디기가 더 쉽다고 한다.
환자는 프리페스트(약)를 지난 주 처방 받았고, 그 후로 줄곧 복용하고 있지만 이 시점에서 별로 효과를 보지 못하고 있고 증세가 호전되기를 절박하게 원한다.

평가: 심각한 증세를 갖고 있는 최근 폐경이 된 52세의 환자

계획: 호르몬 대체 치료에 대해 의논하였고 에스트로겐 용량을 에스트레이스(약) 하루 2밀리그램으로 늘리겠다고 조언했다. 이와 함께 주기적 프로게스테론 사용도 필요하다고 권해 주었고 그 이유는 그녀가 약물중단성 출혈을 보일 것이라고 예상되는 상태이기 때문이다. 약물중단성 출혈은 일시적으로 나타나는 증세라는 것을 확실히 해 두었다.
환자는 에스트레이스 2밀리그램과 프로메트리움 200밀리그램을 12월부터 시작해서 매달 1일부터 12일까지 매일 복용하도록 처방해 주었다. 어떤 출혈이 없는지 계속 관찰하고, 3개월 후에 다시 내원할 것을 지시했다.
환자에게 지난 건강 상태를 보았을 때 이 치료가 얼굴 홍조 증세를 100퍼센트 호전시키지 못할지도 모르겠지만, 시간이 지남에 따라 차차 좋아질 것이라고 말했다. 얼굴 홍조 현상이 나타나는 것과 여성들이 말하는, 증세를 감소시키는 데 도움이 되는 방법들에 대해 이야기를 나누었다.
이 문제가 많이 호전되지 않을 경우, 수면에 대해 도움을 줄 수 있는 이차적 약의 복용에 대해서도 의논하였다. 기록한 대로 3개월 후 다시 내원할 것. 23분간 환자와 보냈고 반 이상의 시간은 상담하는 데 보냈다.

의사 샤론 웰즈

Chart Note ⑦ PATIENT'S RECORDS 환자 진료기록 영문본 【3】

PATIENT'S RECORDS

Ob/Gyn
Name: Jane ××××
DOB: Apr. 11. 1957

Jane is seen in consultation from Jenny Doe regarding severe hot flashes. She is a 52-year-old, white female, whose last menstrual period was over a year ago without any further bleeding since then. She states her hot flushes started at the time of her menses ceased and have become worse, particularly at night. She states she is afraid to lay down because she gets so excessively warm. She does not usually sleep for more than an hour to hour and a half before she gets awakened by a hot flushes, and she will get up and even go outdoors to cool off. The hot flushes are associated with significant perspiration particularly at night. She copes better during the day because when she gets excessively warm, she goes outside to cool off.
The patient was prescribed Prefest last week which she has been on since then but at this point has not seen any benefit and is quite desperate to see some improvement.

ASSESSMENT: Fifty-two-year-old recently menopausal patient with severe symptoms

PLAN: Discussed hormone replacement therapy and advised that we increase her dose of estrogen to Estrace 2 mg daily. Advised that she will need to use a cyclic progesterone with this because she will get withdrawal bleeding, and this will make it in a predictable pattern. Reassured that withdrawal bleeding is a temporary problem.
The patient was given a prescription to use Estrace 2 mg daily and to use prometrium 200 mg daily from the first through the twelfth of the calendar month starting in December. Advised to keep track of any bleeding that occurs and to have follow up after three months.
Advised patient that given her history, this may not control hot flashes 100 percent but hopefully will improve them and that they should improve spontaneously over time. Discussed triggers for hot flushes and some measures that other women find to be helpful to cut their problems. Discussed the addition of a second medication for help with the sleep problem if this does not improve significantly.
Follow up in three months as noted. Twenty-three minutes spent with the patient with over 50 percent in counseling.

Sharon Wells, MD

단어 정리

□ hot flushes	□ 열감(熱感), 피부의 홍조(紅潮)
□ menses(menstruation)	□ 월경
□ perspiration	□ 발한, 땀남
□ menopausal	□ 폐경
□ estrogen	□ 에스트로겐(여포호르몬)
□ progesterone	□ 프로게스테론(황체호르몬)
□ withdrawal bleeding	□ 금단성 출혈
□ prescription	□ 처방
□ trigger	□ 발병, 발생

4) 그 외

Chart Note ① X-RAY REPRORT 엑스레이 보고서 한글본

엑스레이 결과 보고서

date of Service: 12/3/2011

환자이름: ××××

생년월일: 1970년 2월 11일 실시날짜: 2011년 12월 3일

양측 유방암 검사

양측 유방에 치밀한(조밀한) 유선조직이 불규칙하게 분포되어 있다. 의심이 되는 종괴나 석회화는 볼 수 없었다. 방사선 검사결과 악성 소견 없다. 2011년 5월 19일에 실시했던 검사와 비교해 주목할 만한 변화는 없었다.

결론

유방암 결과 음성(정상)

담당의: 김 ××

Chart Note ① X-RAY REPRORT 엑스레이 보고서 영문본

X-RAY REPORT

date of Service: 12/3/2011

Patient Name: ××××
DOB: 2/11/1970

BILATERAL MAMMOGRAM

There is irregularly dense glandular tissue throughout both breasts. There are no suspicious masses or calcifications seen. There is no radiographic evidence of malignancy. There has been no significant change compared with the previous study dated May 19, 2011.

CONCLUSION

Negative mammogram

Dr. ×× Kim

단어 정리

□ bilateral	□ 양측-, 양쪽-의
□ mammogram	□ 유방암 검사
□ dense	□ 조밀-, 치밀-, 진한
□ glandular	□ 샘, 선(腺)
□ tissue	□ 조직
□ calcification	□ 석회화
□ radiographic	□ 방사선상의
□ malignancy	□ 암, 악성
□ negative	□ 음성, 역

Chart Note ② Colposcopy Report 질 확대경검사 보고서 한글본

질 확대경검사 보고서

담당의사: ××××

시술내용
장내시경

시술을 위한 조치사항
올해 10월, 환자는 의미 미결정의 등급이 낮은 상피 질환을 보였고, 아마도 약한 형성이상증이거나 사람 유두종 바이러스에 의한 1등급 자궁목상피내종양일 것이다. 이러한 이유로 우리는 환자에게 질 확대경 검사를 실시할 것이다.

P환자는 21세이고, 출산부 1-0-0-1. 19세에 첫 번째 임신. 환자는 생식기 질환이나 성병 소견 없음.

시술 실시
시술, 위험 요소, 이로운 점, 그리고 가능한 대체 요법 등에 대해 논의하고 환자는 동의서를 작성하였다.

자궁 내시경을 이용하여 질과 자궁 경부를 관찰. 초산용액을 바른 후에, 12시와 1시 방향 사이에서 흰색의 상피조직과 불분명한 주위 조직이 발견되었고, 5시와 6시 방향에서 점적과 불분명한 주변 상태 발견. 자궁경부 후방 쪽까지 퍼져 있으나 원주 모양이고, 자궁경부 전방 밑으로도 발견된다. 뺏속에도 가능성 있다. 12시와 1시 방향, 5시와 6시 방향에서 자궁경 내막 조직 검사를 실시하였다. 병리과에 검사 의뢰 요청.

진단
비정상 자궁암 검사 결과에 대한 질 확대경검사

계획
세포 검사의 병리적 결과를 기다릴 것이다. 심각성의 정도에 따라 동결소작이나 환상투열요법을 권유할 것이다.

Les Perez, MD

LP: KB

D: 12/19/20-
T: 12/20/20-

Chart Note ② Colposcopy Report 질 확대경검사 보고서 영문본

Colposcopy Report

Surgeon: XXXX

PROCEDURE
Colposcopy

INDICATIONS FOR PROCEDURE
In October of this year, patient had a low-grade epithelial lesion of undeterminded significance, probably mild dysplasia or CIN grade 1 with HPV effect. For that reason, we scheduled her for colposcopy.

Patient is 21 years old, para 1-0-0-1. Her age at first pregnancy was 19. She has no history of veneral disease or sexually transmitted infection.

PROCEDURE
After discussion of procedure, risks, benefits, and possible alternatives, patient gave written consent for the procedure.

Speculum was placed in the vagina and cervix brought into view. After applying vinegar, we saw a large transformation zone consisting of white epithelium with mosaic at 12 and 1 o'clock positions and punctation and mosaic at 5 to 6 o'clock. It was more extensive on the posterior cervix, but it went circumferentially and under the anterior cervix, possibly inside the os. Endocervical biopsies were done at 12 and 1 and at 5 and 6 o'clock positions. They were sent separately to pathology.

DIAGNOSIS
Colposcopy for abnormal Pap smear

PLAN
We will await pathology results of biopsies. Then we will recommend either cryocautery or loop electrosurgical excision procedure based on the severity of findings.

Les Perez. MD

LP: KB

D:12/19/20-
T:12/20/20-

단어 정리

☐ epithelial	☐ 상피의
☐ dysplasia	☐ 1. 형성이상(증) 2. 이형성
☐ CIN	☐ 자궁목상피내종양
☐ HPV	☐ 사람 유두종 바이러스
☐ colposcopy	☐ 질 확대경검사
☐ para	☐ 출산
☐ venereal	☐ 성병
☐ speculum	☐ 경, 벌리개
☐ vagina	☐ 질
☐ cervix	☐ 자궁경부
☐ transformation	☐ 전환, 형질전환
☐ epithelium	☐ 상피
☐ mosaic	☐ 불분명하게 주위에 퍼져 있는 상태
☐ circumferencially	☐ 원주 모양으로
☐ endocervical	☐ 자궁경내막
☐ pathology	☐ 병리학
☐ pap smear	☐ 자궁암 검사
☐ electrosurgical excision procedure	☐ 전기외과적절제술

* 참고

para 1-0-0-1이란...

여기서 1과 0이란 숫자는 출산에 관계된 다음과 같은 사실을 보여 줍니다.

full-term baby(만삭되어서 낳은 아기)	1
stillbirth(사산된 경우)	0
artificial abortion(인공 유산)	0
number of child(현재 자녀수)	1

(병원이름)
(주소)

방사선 치료상담

환자이름
생년월일: 1930년 1월 2일

의사 이름
실시 날짜: 200×년 6월 15일

현재 병력: 환자는 72세이고, 2004년 혈관육종으로 감압후궁절제술과 해링턴막대 삽입술을 받았다. 수술 후 방사선 치료를 ××× 병원에서 받았다. 방사선 치료는 일주일에 4회, 그리고 ××× 의사는 척추 T2에서 T8까지를 치료한 것으로 추정하고 있다. 2년 전 척수간 조영상과 단층촬영 결과 이상은 발견되지 않았다. 그러나 지난 달 기침과 객혈 증세를 보였다. **가슴 엑스레이 촬영과 컴퓨터 단층촬영:** 우측 폐문 주위의 덩어리가 가슴 중앙 세로칸까지 확대되어 있고, 후기 폐쇄, 양측 흉막 삼출물과 함께 전방 가슴 세로칸에 1개의 덩어리. **기관지경술 실시:** 우측 상방 기관지구에서 구역 기관지까지 75%의 협착, 우측 하방 기관지구 50% 협착. 우측 상방 기관지구 출혈 오른쪽 흉막 삼출물 배출, 경화증은 세포 진단학상 음성. 우측 기관옆 부위로부터 예비혈관 조직 진단. **종격 내시경:** 혈관 육종 가능성.

과거 병력: 고혈압

사회력: 50세 때 흡연습관

신체검사: 일반: 급성 통증 없는 건강한 남성. 축지성 샘병증 없음. **폐:** 깨끗하다. **심장:** 정상 박동. **복부:** 특정 소견 없음. **사지:** 순환 이상이나 부종 없음. **신경:** 초점성 질환 없음.

평가: 후기 폐쇄 폐렴과 객혈을 동반한 전이성 혈관육종 재발

계획: 증세를 유발하는 종격 질환에 방사선 4000 센티그레이. 화학요법 계획 없음. 방사선 치료의 과정, 위험 요인, 대체 요법 등을 환자와 상의. 예전의 방사선 조사에 의한 이환율의 증가뿐 아니라 척수, 폐, 심장의 장기적 위험 요소에 대해 강조하였다.

Chart Note ③ RADIATION THERAPY CONSULTATION 방사선 치료상담 영문본

College Grove Hospital
4567City College Avenue
Canyon Rim, XY12345

RADIATION THERAPY CONSULTATION

Name: Theodore V. Valdez
Room#499
MR#380780

Requested by: John L. Morris, MD

Date: 6/15/200×

HISTORY OF PRESENT MEDICAL ILLNESS: This is a 72-year-old who underwent decompressive laminectomy and Harrington rod placement in 2004 for angiosarcoma. Postoperative radiation therapy at ××× Hospital: 4 treatments per week, Dr. Davis estimates coverage T2 to T8. Myelogram and CT scan negative 2 years ago. However, developed cough and hemoptysis in past month. **Chest x-ray and CT:** Right perihilar mass extending into mediastinum with multiple central and 1 anterior mediastinal mass with postobstructive infiltrate, bilateral pleural effusion. **Bronchoscopy:** 75% narrowing right upper lobe orifice to subsegments, 50% narrowing right lower lobe orifice. Bleeding at right upper lobe orifice. Draining right pleural effusion and sclerodesis with negative cytology. Preliminary tissue diagnosis from right paratracheal area. **Mediastinoscopy:** Probable angiosarcoma.

PAST MEDICAL HISTORY: Hypertension

SOCIAL HISTORY: 50-year tobacco habit

PHYSICAL EXAMINATION: **General:** Well-developed male in no acute distress. No palpable adenopathy. **Lungs:** Clear. **Heart:** Regular rate and rhythm. **Abdomen:** Unremarkable. **Extremties:** Without circulatory collapse or edema. **Neurologic:** Without focal deficit.

ASSESSMENT: Recurrent metastatic angiosarcoma with postobstructive pneumonitis and hemoptysis.

PLAN: 4000 cGy[1] to symptom-producing mediastinal disease. Initial 1000 cGy[1] at 200 cGy fractions, then oblique off previously irradiated spinal cord ad boost with 250 cGy fractions. No plans for chemotherapy. Discussed radiation therapy procedures, risks, and alternatives with patient, emphasizing possible long-term risks to spinal cord, lung, and heart as well as increased potential for morbidity resulting from prior irradiation. He agrees with treatment as outlined.

단어 정리

□ decompressive	□ 감압
□ laminectomy	□ 후궁절제(술), 고리판절제(술)
□ angiosarcoma	□ 혈관육종
□ myelogram	□ 척수강 조영상
□ hemoptysis	□ 객혈
□ perihilar	□ 폐문주위
□ mediastinum	□ 가슴세로칸, 종격
□ mediastinal	□ 세로칸-, 종격-
□ anterior	□ 앞-, 전방-
□ postobstructive	□ 후기 폐쇄의
□ infiltrate	□ 침윤물
□ bilateral	□ 양측-, 양쪽-
□ bronchoscopy	□ 기관지경술, 기관지보개술
□ lobe orifice	□ 기관지구(~氣管支口)
□ orifice	□ 구멍
□ pleural effusion	□ 흉막삼출
□ subsegments	□ 구역기관지
□ sclerosis	□ 경화(증), 굳음(증)
□ cytology	□ 세포학, 세포진단학
□ preliminary	□ 예비
□ paratracheal	□ 기관옆-
□ mediastinoscopy	□ 종격내시경(법), 세로칸보개검사
□ angiosarcoma	□ 혈관육종
□ palpable	□ 촉지성
□ adenopathy	□ 샘병(증), 선병(증)
□ circulatory	□ 순환-
□ collapse	□ 1. 허탈 2. 붕괴
□ edema	□ 부종
□ focal deficit	□ 초점성 질환
□ metastatic	□ 1. 전아- 2. 전이성-
□ angiosarcoma	□ 혈관육종

□ pneumonitis	□ 폐렴
□ hemoptysis	□ 객혈
□ cGy: centigray	□ (1 rad) 방사선의 단위(unit of radiation)
□ chemotherapy	□ 화학요법
□ morbidity	□ 이환률
□ irradiation	□ 방사선 조사

Chart Note ④ DISCHARGE SUMMARY 퇴원 보고서 한글본

Evans, Cornelia Elizabeth
97-32-11
July 16, 200×

퇴원 보고서

입원일: 200×년 6월 14일 퇴원일: 200×년 7월 15일

현 병력: 이 19세의 미산부(임신한 적이 없는) 여성은 200×년 6월 14일 병원에 왔고 당시 화씨 102도의 열, 왼쪽 하복부 통증, 질분비물, 변비 그리고 왼쪽 부속기 종양(덩어리) 압통이 있었다. 환자 자신의 병력이나 가족병력에 특이사항 없다. 현재의 통증은 내원하기 2~3주전에 시작되었다. 그녀의 생리는 불규칙하고 마지막 월경은 200×년 5월 30일 시작되어 6일간 지속되었다. 환자는 과거 피임약을 복용하였으나 성생활을 하지 않기 때문에 더 이상 복용하지 않게 되었다.

신체검사: 환자는 신체가 잘 발달되고 영양상태가 양호하고 문제가 심각하지 않은 것으로 보였다. 이상에 대해 양성 반응을 나타내는 육체적인 부위는 배와 골반에만 한정되어 있다. 그녀의 복부는 약간 팽만되어 있고, 특별히 왼쪽 하복부에 압통을 느낀다. 골반 진찰 결과, 자궁경부는 움직일 때 압통을 느끼고, 자궁은 정상 크기이며, 후굴되어 있다. 자궁 부속기에 낭종이 있으며 4~5센티미터쯤의 크기이다. 직장 검사결과는 이상 없다.

내원시 진단
1. 골반염증성 질환 가능성
2. 자궁외 임신 가능성 제외

내원시 검사 자료: 헤모글로빈 8.8, 적혈구 용적율 26.5, 백혈구수 8100. 침전율 시간당 100밀리미터. 소변검사 정상. 전해질 정상. 가슴 엑스레이 정상.

병원 치료: 처음에 2일간 세파로틴 2그램 정맥주사 매 6시간마다 주었고, 카나마이신 0.5그램, 근육주사를 하루에 두 번 투여했고 환자의 상태가 호전되었다. 그녀의 통증은 감소되었고, 아침에는 체온도 정상으로 떨어졌고, 저녁때 다시 101도로 올라갔다. 혈액검사를 재실시하였고 그 결과 헤모글로빈 7.8 적혈구 용적율 23.5이다. 임신 검사결과는 음성이다(임신이 아님). 입원 후 2일째 되는 날 밤에는 104도로 올라갔다. 환자는 아이소니아지드(약) 하루에 300밀리그램, 에탐뷰톨 600밀리그램 하루 두 번, 리팜핀 하루에 600밀리그램의 결핵 치료를 받기 시작했다. 그녀는 수술 후 6일째 되는 때 열이 없어졌고 200×년 7월 15일 호전된 상태로 퇴원하였다. 1주일 후에 재진을 할 것이다.

외과적 시술: 동결절편의 그물막 생검; 표본 배양

퇴원시 진단: 생식기 결핵

____
담당의사 서명

Chart Note ④ DISCHARGE SUMMARY 퇴원 보고서 영문본

Evans, Cornelia Elizabeth
97-32-11
July 16, 200×

DISCHARGE SUMMARY

ADMISSIN DATE: June 14, 200× DISCHARGE DATE: July 15, 200×

HISTORY OF PRESENT ILLNESS: This 19-year-old female nulligravida was admitted to the hospital on June 14, 200×, with fever of 102°, left lower quadrant pain, vaginal discharge, constipation, and a tender left adnexal mass. Her past history and family history were unremarkable. Present pain had started 2 to 3 weeks prior to admission. Her periods were irregular, with the latest period starting on May 30, 200×, and lasting for 6 day. She had taken contraceptive pills in the past but had stopped because she was not sexually active.

PHYSICAL EXAMINATION: She appeared well developed and well nourished and in mild distress. The only positive physical findings were limited to the abdomen and pelvis. Her abdomen was mildly distended, and it was tender, especially in the left lower quadrant. At pelvic examination, the cervix was tender on motion, and the uterus was of normal size, retroverted. There was a tender cystic mass, about 4 to 5 cm, in the left adnexa, Rectal examination was negative.

ADMITTING DIAGNOSES
1. Probable pelvic inflammatory disease(PID)
2. Rule out ectopic pregnancy

LABORATORY DATA ON ADMISSION: Hemoglobin 8.8, hematocrit 26.5, WBC 8100. Sedimentation rate 100 mm in 1 hour. Urinalysis normal. Electrolytes normal. Chest x-ray negative.

HOSPITAL COURSE AND TREATMENT: Initially, she was given cephalothin 2 g IV q.6h. and kanamycin 0.5g IM b.i.d. Over the next 2days, the patient's condition improved. Her pain decreased, and her temperature came down to normal in the morning and spiked to 101° in the evening. Repeat CBS showed hemoglobin 7.8, hematocrit 23.5. The pregnancy test was negative. On the 2nd night following admission, she spiked to 104°. The patient was started on antituberculosis treatment consisting of isoniazid 300mg per day, ethambutol 600mg b.i.d., and rifampin 600mg daily. She became afebrile on the 6th postoperative day and was discharged on Jury 15, 200×, in good condition. She will be seen in the office in 1 week.

SURGICAL PROCEDURES: Biopsy of omentum for frozen section; culture specimens

DISCHARGE DIAGNOSIS: Genital tuberculosis

Dr. signature

단어 정리

□ nulligravida	□ 미산부
□ adnexal	□ 부속기
□ contraceptive	□ 피임제
□ pelvis	□ 골반
□ distended	□ 팽창된
□ cervix	□ 자궁경부
□ uterus	□ 자궁
□ cystic	□ 낭-, 낭종-
□ rectal	□ 직장-, 곧창자-
□ inflammatory	□ 염증-
□ ectopic	□ 딴곳-, 전위-, 편위-
□ lymph	□ 림프
□ Sedimentation	□ 침전, 침강
□ CBC(Cmplete Blood Count)	□ 혈액검사
□ PID(Pelvic Inflammatory Disease)	□ 골반 염증성 질환
□ hematocrit	□ 적혈구용적율
□ urinalysis	□ 요검사
□ electrolytes	□ 전해질
□ afebrile	□ 무열성(無熱性)의
□ postoperative	□ 수술후
□ biopsy	□ 생검, 조직 검사
□ omentum	□ 그물막, 망
□ genital	□ 1. 생식- 2. 생식기(관)-
□ tuberculosis	□ 결핵
□ IV	□ 정맥 주사
□ IM	□ 근육 주사
□ frozen section	□ 동결절편

4. 경과 보고서(Progress Note)

경과 보고서란 환자의 초진 시 작성하는 의료기록지와 달리 그 이후의 모든 진료 내용을 기록한 것이다. 여기에는 의료진이 환자의 상태에 대한 자세한 내용, 치료 내용, 외래 진료, 입원 상황 등이 포함된다.

여러 가지 데이터, 치료 계획, 또 치료에 따른 변화 관찰 및 검토 등도 상세히 기술된다.

경과기록은 의사의 경향, 어떤 내용을 중점적으로 기록할 것인지 등에 따라 여러 가지 다양한 형식으로 기록될 수 있으나 앞서 말했듯이 가장 흔하게 쓰이는 형식은 SOAP 형식으로 주관적 관찰(Subjective), 객관적 관찰(Objective), 치료시행(Assessment), 그리고 치료계획(Plan) 등의 순으로 기록한다.

특별히 치료와 치료 과정을 시간적 순서(chronological sequence)에 따라 주로 의사와 간호사가 기록하며 내용으로는 치료와 약의 사용, 그에 따른 변화, 검사결과 등이 있다. 이러한 내용을 바탕으로 의료진은 환자의 상태를 비교·검토하고, 향후 치료계획에 적용하여, 좀 더 효과적인 결정을 할 수 있게 된다.

이러한 기록은 환자의 치료 내용과 과정에 따라 병원 내 여러 분야에서 동시에 활용될 수 있으며, 이제 모든 내용이 전자화되어 있어 접근이 매우 편리하게 되었다.

의사는 환자를 진료할 때마다 매번 경과 기록을 작성해야만 하는데, 이 기록은 치료에만 쓰이는 것이 아니라, 필요에 따라 법적 효력을 갖게 되며, 또한 의료비 청구에도 필요한 기록이 된다. 따라서 그 내용은 정확하고, 완전하고, 세부적 사항까지도 포함하여야 한다.

Progress Record ① Progress Record 경과 보고서 한글본

××× 병원 경과 기록지 S = 객관적 관찰내용 O = 주관적 관찰내용 A = 진찰/진단 P = 계획 E = 평가	이름 환자 번호 생년월일 차트 번호

날짜/시간	문제/통제	증세, 데이터, 시간 그 외 모든 내용
		의사 서명

Progress Record ① Progress Record 경과 보고서 영문본

×××Medical Center

Progress Record

S = Subjective
O = Objective
A = Assessment/Impression
P = Plan
E = Evaluation

Chart number

NAME

CONSUMER NUMBER

DATE OF BIRTH

DATE/ TIME	PROBLEM/ DISCIPLINE	Sign, data, and time all entries
		Dr.'s signature

IV. 환자동의서 (Patient Consent Form)

Consent ① Patient Consent Form 치과 환자동의서 한글본

xxxx
치과

xxxx 치과
주소
전화번호

환자동의서

나는 제 자신의 건강 정보가 보호받아야 하며, 저에게 데이터의 기밀성에 대한 권리가 있다는 것을 이해합니다. 저는 또한 이 동의서에 서명함으로써 의료기관이 다음과 같은 일을 수행하는 데 저의 건강 정보가 사용되고 공개되는 것에 동의하게 됨을 이해합니다.

- 치료(본인의 치료에 일환으로 행해지는 다른 의료기관에서의 직접적 또는 간접적 치료 포함)
- 제3자로부터의 의료비 수거(예: 본인의 의료 보험사)
- 의료기관의 일상적인 행정상 운영

나는 나의 보호받고 있는 건강정보 사용과 공개, 그에 따른 나의 권리 등에 대한 내용에 대해 설명을 들었고, 그것에 대해 검토할 수 있는 기회도 있었고, 문서화된 내용도 제공받았습니다.
나는 귀하가 때에 따라 이 동의서의 유효기간을 변경할 수 있는 권리가 있다는 것을 이해하며, 가장 최근의 정보를 위해 언제라도 연락할 수 있다는 것을 알고 있습니다.

나는 이 동의서의 파기를 언제든지 서면으로 취소할 수 있다는 것을 이해하고 있습니다.
그러나 이미 앞서 이 동의서의 효력 아래에서 일어난 일들에 대해서 동의서의 파기는 무관합니다.

환자 이름 ____
환자와의 관계 ____________________________________

참조: 다음 병원 방문때 날짜와 서명란에 기입하실 수 있습니다.

서명 날짜 20_______년_______월_______일
서명:
____

Consent ① Patient Consent Form 치과 환자동의서 영문본

XXXX
DENTAL
GROUP

XXXX Dental Center
address
phone

PATIENT CONSENT FORM

I understand that I have certain right to privacy regarding my protected health information.
I understand that by signing this consent I authorize you to use and disclose my protected health information to carry out:

- Treatment(including direct or indirect treatment by other healthcare providers involved in my treatment)
- Obtaining payment from third party payers(e.g. my insurance company)
- The day-to day healthcare operations of your practice

I have also been informed of, and given the right to review and secure a copy, which contains a more complete description of the uses and disclosures of my protected health information.
I understand that you reserve the right to change the terms of this notice form time to time and that I may contact you at time to obtain the most current copy of this notice.

I understand that I may revoke this consent, in writing, at any time. However, any use or disclosure that occurred prior to the date I revoke this consent is not affected.

Patient Name ________________________________

Relationship To Patient ________________________

NOTE: You will have an opportunity to DATE and SIGN this form during your next visit

Signed this ________day of ____________, 20 ____

Signature:

____

단어 정리

□ privacy	□ 사적(私的)(개인적) 비밀, 내밀(內密)

* medical privacy 의료 프라이버시, 개인 의료기록 보호

□ disclose	□ (비밀 따위)를 폭로하다, 노출시키다
□ treatment	□ 치료; 치료법(for)
□ day-to day	□ 나날의(daily)
□ operation	□ 운영
□ term	□ 기간, 기한, 약정 기간(기일)
□ revoke	□ …을 취소하다, 폐지하다, 무효로 하다
□ disclosure	□ 발표, 공개; (기업의) 정보 공개
□ affect	□ …에 영향을 미치다

Consent ② Medical Consent Form 진료동의서 한글본

의료동의서

모두 기입한 후에만 효력을 발생할 수 있습니다.
참가자 성명(정자로 기입): ______________________________
부모 혹은 보호자 성명(정자로 기입): ______________________________

내 자신, 혹은 배우자, 나의 자녀들 중 누구라도 어떤 상황에서 사고를 당하거나 상해를 입었을 경우 내가 현장에 없거나, 또는 치료에 동의할 수 없는 경우

1.	나는 어떤 병원, 의사, 혹은 그 병원 소속 의사들이 필요하다고 생각하거나, 권고가 있을 때 나 자신, 내 배우자, 혹은 나의 아이들 중 누구라도 의료적 보호와 간호, 치료를 받는 것에 자발적으로 동의합니다.
2.	나는 의료적 보호, 간호, 치료 등을 제공해 줄 것을 병원 의료진에게 허락합니다.
3.	나는 의료적 보호, 간호, 치료에 대한 비용에 대해 손해를 입히지 않고 공정한 지불을 할 것에 동의합니다.

나는, 의료진과 적법한 자격이 부여된 치과 의사 등의 적합한 관리 하에 엑스레이 검사, 마취, 그리고 의료적, 외과적 진단과 시술 등을 제공하는 것에 서명하고, 수락합니다. 나는 이렇게 미리 병의 진단, 치료, 병원의 보호 등에 대해 동의함으로써, 전술한 의사가 판단하고 권유하는 모든 치료의 제공을 허락하고 그에게 권한을 부여하는 것입니다. 이는 환자에게 치료를 하기 전에 아래 서명자에게 연락을 취하겠지만 서명자와 연락이 되지 않는 상황이라 할지라도 위의 치료가 지연되어서는 안 된다는 것을 의미합니다.

응급시 연락처:

성명	관계	전화번호

부모 서명/보호자:______________________날짜:______________

가장 최근에 치료받은 의사:

성명	전화번호	마지막 진료일

보험 가입자	보험 등록자 번호	보험 등록자 성명	보험 등록자 생년월일
보험 가입자 주소	보험 가입자 전화 #	등록자와 가입자의 관계	등록자 전화 #

Consent ② Medical Consent Form 진료동의서 영문본

MEDICAL CONSENT FORM

Only COMPLETELY FILLED IN forms will be accepted.
NAME OF PARTICIPANT (printed): ______________________________
NAME OF PARENT OR GUARDIAN (printed): ______________________________

In the event of accident or injury to myself, my spouse or and any child of mine(or in the event of illness of myself, my spouse or any child of mine while participating in any activity under circumstances where I am physically unable to consent or am not present

1. I hereby voluntarily consent the furnishing to myself, my spouse or any of my said children of such medical care, attention and treatment by any hospital, physician or physicians as such hospital, physician or physicians may deem necessary or advisable.
2. I authorize any medical staffs of this Hospital to consent to such medical care, attention or treatment.
3. I agree to pay the reasonable cost of such medical care, attention or treatment and to indemnify and hold free and harmless of and from any and all liability for such cost.

I, the undersigned, do hereby authorize and consent to any x-ray examination, anesthetic, medical or surgical diagnosis or procedure rendered under the general of specific supervision of any member of the medical staff or of a dentist licensed under the provisions. It is understood that this authorization is given in advance of any specific diagnosis, treatment or hospital care being required but is given to provide authority and power to render care which the aforementioned physician in the exercise of his best judgment may deem advisable. It is understood that effort shall be made to contact the undersigned prior to rendering treatment to the patient, but that any of the above treatment will not be withheld if the undersigned cannot be reached.

IN CASE OF EMERGENCY CALL:

NAME	RELATIONSHIP	PHONE NUMBER

SIGNATURE OF PARENT/GUARDIAN:______________________DATE:______________

PHYSICIAN WHO CONDUCTED YOUR MOST RECENT PHYSICAL EXAMINATION:

NAME	PHONE NUMBER	DATE OF LAST EXAM

Insurance Carrier	Policy Number	Policy Holder's Name	Policy Holder's Date of Birth
Insurance Carrier Address	Insurance Carrier Phone #	Policy Holder's Relation to Participant	Policy Holder Phone #

단어 정리

□ injury	□ 부상, 상해
□ spouse	□ 배우자
□ voluntarily	□ 자발적으로, 임의로
□ circumstance	□ (주변의) 상황, 환경, 사정
□ furnish	□ (필요한 것)을 공급하다, 제공하다, 주다
□ indemnify	□ (손해에 대하여) …에게 보장하다
□ harmless	□ 피해가 없는
□ liability	□ (…의/…할) 책임(이 있음)
□ provision	□ 〈법률〉 조항, 규정
□ aforemention	□ 전술한, 전기(前記)한
□ undersigned (the ~)	□ 〈단·복수 양용〉 서명자
□ withheld	□ withhold 의 과거형. …을 주는 것을 보류하다

Consent ③ Medical and Emergency Information 응급동의서 한글본

진료와 응급시 환자 정보

이름: ______________________________ 성별____(남)____(여)

주소: ____

____

전화번호: ______________(집)______________(직장) 생년월일______________

환자 그리고 그/그녀의 부모는 아래 질문에 가능한 한 정확하게 모든 질문에 답하셔야만 합니다.

해당사항을 기록하세요(자세한 내용을 아래에 기록하세요)

만성 질병		알레르기 반응	
천식, 혹은 다른 호흡기 질환		약	
당뇨 혹은 저혈당증		벌에 쏘임/벌레 물림	
혈우병, 혹은 출혈성 질환		음식들	
순환기 혹은 심장 문제		그 외, 만약 심각하다면	
간질			

자세히 기록하세요: ____

____

____

마지막 파상풍 주사 접종 날짜: ______________ 혈액형:______________

만약 현재 복용하는 약이 있다면: ______________________________

위의 성명 란에 기록한 사람에게 어떤 병리적 증세가 있나요?

만약 있다면, 설명하세요:

____

____

____

필요한 사항들을 다 기입했는지 확인해 주세요

Consent ③ Medical and Emergency Information 응급동의서 영문본

MEDICAL AND EMERGENCY INFORMATION

NAME: ______________________________ SEX____(M)____(F)

ADDRESS: ______________________________

____

TELEPHONE: ______________(R)______________(B) DATE OF BIRTH______________

THE PATIENT AND HIS OR HER PARENTS MUST RESPOND TO THE FOLLOWING QUESTIONS AS ACCURATELY AND COMPLETELY AS POSSIBLE.

Please check those that apply(Provide necessary details below)

CHRONIC AILMENTS		ALLERGIES	
ASTHMA, OR OTHER RESPIRATORY PROBLEMS		MEDICATION	
DIABETES OR HYPOGLYCEMIA		BEE STINGS/INSECT BITES	
HEMOPHILIA, OR OTHER BLEEDING PROBLEMS		FOODS	
CIRCULATORY OR HEART PROBLEMS		OTHERS, IF SIGNIFICANT	
EPILEPSY			

DETAILS: ______________________________

____

____

DATE OF LAST TETANUS SHOT: ______________BLOOD TYPE: ______________

CURRENT MEDICATIONS IF ANY: ______________________________

DOES THE ABOVE NAMED INDIVIDUAL HAVE ANY MEDICAL CONDITION?

IF YES, PLEASE EXPLAIN:

____

____

____

PLEASE MAKE SURE YOU HAVE FILLED IN ALL THE NECESSARY INFORMATION

단어 정리

□ (R)=Residence	□ 집
□ (B)=Business	□ 직장
□ (M)=Male	□ 남성
□ (F)=Female	□ 여성
□ asthma	□ 천식
□ respiratory problems	□ 호흡기 문제
□ hypoglycemia	□ 저혈당(低血糖)(증)
□ hemophilia	□ 혈우병(血友病)
□ bleeding problems	□ 출혈 문제
□ circulatory	□ 순환기의
□ heart problems	□ 심장 문제
□ epilepsy	□ 〈병리〉 간질
□ bee sting	□ 벌에 쏘임
□ insect bites	□ 벌레 물림
□ significantg	□ 중요한, 심각한
□ tetanus	□ 〈병리〉 파상풍; 파상풍균
□ blood type	□ 혈액형

산부인과

의사의 외과적 수술 및 시술동의서

날짜:________________ 시간:____________________오전/오후

1. 나는 아래 수술 또는 시술을 시행하는 것에 동의합니다.
   (전문용어): ____
   환자 성명____
   (나 자신 혹은 환자 이름)
   수술 또는 시술의 목적은(비전문가적인 서술): ______________________________
   ______________________________이고 시술자는 (성명______________)와 그가 지명한 보조자들.

2. 나에게 수술 또는 시술의 성격, 이로운 점과 위험 요소들, 부작용의 가능성과 대체 치료법 등에 대한 설명이 이루어졌습니다.

3. 좋은 결과를 기대할 수 있다는 것에 대해 설명을 들었습니다. 그러나 다음과 같은 몇 가지 부작용이나 영향들이 일어날 수도 있습니다: 출혈, 감염, 근접한 조직이나 기관의 손상, 부종, 통증, 봉합반응, 치유 지연, 흉터, 마취 혹은 약에 대한 부작용, 재발, 추가적 수술, 드물게 마비 혹은 사망; 그 외:____
   ____

4. 결과에 대해서 어떤 보장이나 확신도 주어지지 않았습니다.

5. 나는 의사에게 수술이나 시술 중에 의사가 적합하다고 생각하고, 권고하는 다른 추가적인 수술이나 시술을 시행하는 것에도 동의합니다.

6. 나는 이 수술이나 시술에 필요하다고 생각되는 마취 요법 사용에 동의합니다.

7. 나는 다음 사항을 제외하고는 알레르기 반응이나 과민성 반응은 없습니다.____________________

나는 내용을 모두 읽었고 이해하며, 복사본도 받았습니다.

______________	____
증인 서명	환자, 환자의 부모 혹은 환자 대신 적법하게 서명할 수 있는 자(정자로 기입)
______________	____
의사 서명	환자, 환자의 부모 혹은 환자 대신 적법하게 서명할 수 있는 자의 서명

환자에게 복사

Consent ④ Physician's Surgery & Procedure Consent Form (Ob/Gyn) 영문본

Ob/Gyn

PHYSICIAN'S SURGERY & PROCEDURE CONSENT FORM

Date:________________ Time:____________________a.m./p.m.

1. I consent to the performance of the following operation or procedure.
   (technical name): ____
   upon ____
   (myself or name patient)
   The purpose of this operation or procedure is(lay language): ______________________
   ____________________and will be performed by______________________
   and whomever(s)he may designate as assistants.
2. The nature and purpose of the operation or procedure, the benefits and risks of the operation or procedure, the possibilities of complications and the alternatives to this operation or procedure, their risks and benefits have been explained to me.
3. It has been explained to me that a satisfactory result is expected, but that the following are some of the complications or effects that could or may occur: bleeding, infection, damage to adjacent tissues or organs, swelling, pain, suture reaction, delayed healing, scarring, anesthesia or medication reaction, recurrence, additional operations, and in rare instances paralysis or death; other:____
   ____
4. No guarantee or assurance has been given by anyone about the results that may be obtained.
5. I consent to the doctors performing whatever different or additional operations or procedures they deem necessary or advisable during the course of the operation or procedure.
6. I consent to administration of such anesthetics as may be considered necessary or advisable for this operation or procedure.
7. I do not have allergies or intolerance to anything except______________________

I have read and understand the content of this form and have received a copy.

____________________	______________________________________
Witness to signing	Patient, parent or person authorized to sign for patient(please print)
____________________	______________________________________
Physician's signature	Signature of patient, parent or person authorized to sign for patient

COPY TO PATIENT

단어 정리

☐ lay	☐ 비전문가의, 문외한의, 일반인의
☐ designate	☐ 지명을 받은
☐ operation	☐ 수술
☐ procedure	☐ (의학적인) 처치, 시술
☐ benefits	☐ 이로움
☐ risks	☐ 위험, 손해(손상)을 입을 우려
☐ satisfactory	☐ 만족한
☐ bleeding	☐ 출혈
☐ infection	☐ 감염
☐ damage	☐ 손상
☐ adjacent	☐ 근접(인접)한, 붙어 있는
☐ tissues	☐ 조직
☐ organs	☐ 기관
☐ swelling	☐ 부종
☐ pain	☐ 통증
☐ suture reaction	☐ 봉합 반응
☐ delayed healing	☐ 치유 지연
☐ scarring	☐ 흉터
☐ anesthesia or medication reaction	☐ 마취 혹은 약물 반응
☐ recurrence	☐ 재발
☐ additional operations	☐ 추가 수술
☐ rare instances	☐ 드문 경우들
☐ paralysis	☐ 마비
☐ possibilities	☐ 가능성
☐ complications	☐ 부작용
☐ alternatives	☐ 대체 요법들
☐ guarantee	☐ 보장
☐ assurance	☐ 확신
☐ intolerance	☐ (음식물·약에 대한) 과민성

의료적/외과적 시술동의서

◉ 병원전문 과목 ◉ 주소 ◉ 전화번호

나(혹은 저의 대리인, 예를 들어 환자 보호자), (환자의 이름)________________________는 의료적/외과적 시술이 (담당의사명)________________________과 그 의료진들, 의료보조자들에 의해 시행되는 것에 동의한다. 시술시 한 명 또는 그 이상의 의사가 시술을 하거나 마무리할 수 없을 때 자격이 있는 의사가 할 수 있다.

의료적/외과적 시술 (시술명)____________________을 제시하며, (병명)___________________의 진단/치료이다. 시술은 나에게 이해할 수 있는 언어로 설명되었다. 그리고 설명은 다음과 같은 사항을 포함한다:

- 시술의 내용과 범위
- 시술에서 가장 자주 일어나는 위험요인들, 그리고 초래될 수 있는 심각한 결과들, 다음과 같은 내용이 포함된다. ____
  ____
- 통증, 상처, 감염 등의 일반적 위험요인들
- 시술의 이로움
- 정상 활동이 안 되거나 요양시설에 있어야 하는 기간의 정도, 만약 있다면__________________
- 가능한 대체 요법의 사용이나 혹은 시술을 받지 않을 경우 이로운 점과 해로운 점

나는 시술에 대하여 질문할 수 있는 기회가 주어졌고, 내가 만족할 만한 대답을 들었다. 나는 다른 의사와 이 문제를 상의해도 무방하고, 상의할 수도 있다.

나는 의사가 나의 증세나 진단에 적합하다고 판단되거나 부가적으로 시술이 필요하다고 판단되면 시술을 해도 좋다고 허락한다.

만약 시술하는 중에 예상치 않았던 상황이 생겨서 병원으로 호송되거나, 부가적인 시술, 또는 마취나 수혈이 필요한 수술을 하게 되면 나를 대신해서 의사가 이런 사항을 결정하는 것에 동의한다.

나는 의학이나 수술이 항상 동일하고 정확한 과학이 아니라는 것을 이해하며, 나는 이 시술의 결과에 어떤 보장도 되지 않는다는 것을 알고 있다.

나는 의사와 그 외 의사가 지목하는 의료진, 협력자, 보조자 등이 시술에 참여하는 것을 허락하며, 의사의 분별력에 따라 다음과 같은 경우 신체 조직의 폐기나 신체의 일부를 제거하는 등의 시술을 할 수 있다는 것도 수락한다. (만약 있다면):____

다음 페이지 2에서 계속

Consent ④ Consent to Medical/Surgical Office Procedure 영문본 【1】

Consent to Medical/Surgical Office Procedure

◉ Office Practice Name ◉ Address ◉ Telephone

I(or my authorize representative, i.e., parent guardian), ____________________________, consent to the medical/surgical procedures outlined below to be performed by ____________________________ and his/her staff, associates, or assistants whom the physician(s)performing the procedure may assign designated responsibilities. In the event one or more of the physicians is unable to perform or complete the procedure, a qualified substitute physician will perform or complete the procedure.

The propose medical/surgical procedure is ____________________________ for the diagnosis/treatment of ________________. The procedure has been explained to me in terms that I understand. The explanation included:

- The nature and extent of the procedure to be performed
- The most frequently occurring risks of the procedure involved, and those risks which are unlikely to occur but which may involve serious consequences, include but are not necessarily limited to the following: ____
  ____
- General risks which may include pain, scarring, bleeding and infection
- The benefits of the procedure
- The estimated period of incapacity or convalescence, if any
- The risks and benefits of any reasonable alternatives to this procedure including having no treatment at all

I was given the opportunity to ask any questions I have regarding the procedure and I have had those questions answered to my satisfaction.

I understand that I may consult or could have consulted with another physician about this procedure.

I understand that I have the right to refuse any medical/surgical treatment recommended at any time prior to its performance.

I authorized my physician to perform such additional procedures which in his/her judgment are incidentally necessary or appropriate to carry out my diagnosis/treatment.

If any unforeseen condition arises during this procedure which requires transportation to a hospital, additional procedures, operation or medication including anesthesia and blood transfusions, I further request and authorize my physician to do whatever he/she deems advisable on my behalf.

I am aware that the practice of medicine and surgery is not and exact science, and I acknowledge that no guarantees have been made to me concerning the results of this procedure.

I authorize the physician performing the procedure, of his/her staff, associate, or assistant to whom the physician may assign the responsibility, to use his or her discretion in disposing of or using any tissue or body parts that may be removed during the procedure set forth above, subject to the following condition(if any):____

continued page 2

나는 훈련 중에 있는 의사가 시술 중에 참관할 수 있다는 것을 수락한다. 의료 기구회사의 대표나 기술자가 시술에 참관할 수 있다는 것도 수락한다. 의료적인 사진은 의료, 과학, 또 교육적 목적으로 쓰일 수 있으며, 나의 신상은 나타나지 않는다.
나는 위의 사항을 읽었고(읽어 주었고), 충분히 이해한다.
더욱이 나의 모든 시술에 대한 질문들, 걱정, 수반되는 위험요소들, 이로운 점과 대체 방법들에 대해 만족할 만큼 들었고, 나는 위에 논의된 시술을 의사가 시행하는 것에 동의한다.

환자 이름 약자______________/날짜_____________(아래 이름 전부를 서명해 주세요)

진정 진통 [의식 있는 상태에서 진정 진통]

나는 권고받은 대로 진정 진통요법 적용을 받게 된다는 것을 이해한다. 진정 상태의 이로움은 시술 동안 편안하게 해주는 것이다. 모든 진정 요법의 적용은 위험 요소를 갖고 있다는 사실이 나에게 설명되었다. 나는 시술이나 진정 요법에 대한 어떠한 보장이나 약속을 받을 수 없다는 것을 이해한다. 진정 진통요법은 합병증을 유발할 수 있으며 부적합한 진정 요법, 약에 대한 반응, 감염의 가능성, 정맥의 혈관에 출혈이나 상해 등이 포함된다. 좀 더 심한 합병증에는 그보다 더 심각한 결과를 가져올 수 있는 호흡의 저하, 심장 문제 등 심지어 사망까지도 가져올 수 있다. 진정 요법을 적용하지 않는 경우를 포함해 다른 대체 요법에 대해 설명을 들었다.
나는 위의 정보에 대해 다 읽었고 이해한다.
더욱이 진정 요법 적용, 수반되는 위험 요소, 이로운 점, 대체 요법 등에 대한 나의 질문이나 걱정에 대해 모두 답해 주었다는 것을 보증한다. 나는 진정상태가 아직 내 몸 안에 남아 있으므로 24시간 내에 자동차를 운전하거나 기계를 작동하거나, 어떤 법적 결정을 하지 않을 것에 대해 동의한다. 나는 나의 담당의사 그리고/혹은 자격이 있는 자의 진정작용 요법 적용하는 것에 동의한다.

환자 이름_____________/날짜______________(전체 이름 서명)

____ ____________________

환자 서명/공증인/보호자 생년월일

____

증인 서명

____

날짜/시간

나는 동의자에게 이 문서의 내용에 대해서 설명하였습니다. 나의 견해로는 동의자가 논의된 모든 문제들을 충분히 이해하였다고 봅니다.

____

의사 서명

Consent ④ Consent to Medical/Surgical Office Procedure 영문본 【2】

I authorize that a physician in training may participate in my care; a representative or technician from a medical device company may be present at the procedure; medical photography may be utilized for medical, scientific, or educational purposes, provided my identity is not revealed in the photo or text.

I acknowledge that I have read(or had read to me)and fully understand the above information. Furthermore, I certify that all my questions and concerns regarding the procedure, ist attendant risks, benefits and alternatives have been explained to my satisfaction, I hereby authorize my physician to perform the above discussed procedure.

Patient Initials ________________/Date________________(Full signature required below)

Sedative Analgesia [Conscious Sedation]

I understand the administration of sedative analgesia is recommended. The benefit of the sedation is greater comfort throughout the procedure. It has been explained to me tat all forms of sedation involve some risks. I understand that no guarantees or promises can be made concerning the results of my procedure or the sedation technique administered. Complications with sedative analgesia can occur and include: inadequate sedation, drug reaction, the possibility of infection, bleeding or injury to blood vessels at the intravenous site. More severe complications could include depression of respiration and heart problems tat could lead to serious consequences, including even loss of life. Alternatives to sedation include no sedation at all, and have been explained to me.

I acknowledge that I have read(or had read to me)and understand the above information on sedative analgesia. Furthermore, I certify that all my questions and concerns regarding the administration of conscious sedation, its attendant risks, benefits and alternatives have been explained to my satisfaction. I agree not to drive a car operate machinery or make any legal decision within 24 hours as the effect of sedation may remain in my system for this period of time. I hereby authorize my physician and/or individuals qualified to do so, to administer this analgesic.

Patient Initials________________/Date________________(Full signature required below)

______________________________________ ______________________

Patient's Signature/Power of Attorney/Guardian Date of Birth

____

Witness to Signature

____

Date/Time

I verify that I have explained the information contained in this document to the patient or person giving consent. It is my opinion that the person granting consent has fully understood all subjects discussed.

____

Physician Signature

병원명 조영제 주사동의서	이름 환자 번호 생년월일

귀하는 조영제 주입이 필요한 검사를 할 예정입니다.(엑스레이 염색제) 조영제는 작은 정맥 주사로 주입될 것입니다. 이 주사는 검사를 시행하고 판독하는 데 필요합니다. 조영제 없이는 검사결과를 정확히 알 수 없고, 진단에 충분한 자료가 되지 못할 것입니다.
조영제는 자주 사용되며, 일상적인 것이라고 볼 수 있습니다. 250명 중에 한 명에서 500명 중에 한 명 정도 비율로 심하지 않은 부작용이 나타날 수 있습니다. 약한 부작용에는 재채기, 두드러기, 목이 따끔거림, 눈물이 많이 나거나, 매슥거림 등이 있습니다. 이러한 증세는 잠시 나타날 수 있고, 저절로 없어지거나, 항히스타민제 복용으로 회복시킬 수 있습니다.
심각한 증세(혈압의 저하, 호흡 곤란, 심장 마비, 의식 불명, 신장 부전 등)는 5,000명 중에 1명 비율로 나타날 수 있습니다.
사망은 75,000명 중에 1명 비율 정도로 나타날 수 있습니다.
드물게, 조영제가 혈관에서 누출될 수도 있습니다. 이는 심각한 조직 손상을 가져올 수 있고, 교정을 위해 수술을 해야 할 수도 있습니다. 영구적 흉터 그리고/혹은 신경 혹은 근육 손상도 누출이나 수술의 결과로 일어날 수 있습니다.

저희가 최선의 배려를 제공할 수 있도록 다음 질문에 대답해 주십시오.

1. 나이: ______________
2. 알레르기 증세가 있나요(약물, 환경, 그리고 음식 알레르기)? 네 아니오
   만약 있다면 기록하세요: ______________
3. 예전에 조영제 알레르기 반응이 나타난 경험이 있으십니까(엑스레이 염색제)? 네 아니오
   만약 있다면 어떤 종류: ______________
4. 다음과 같은 건강 문제나 질병이 있으십니까?

_______ 천식	_______ 심장질환	_______ 고혈압
_______ 당뇨	_______ 다발 골수종	_______ 겸상적혈구병
_______ 크롬친화세포종	_______ 신장 질환	_______ 적혈구증가증

   그 외: ______________
5. 임신중이십니까? 네 아니오 모유 수유하십니까? 네 아니오
6. 현재 복용 중인 약을 기록하세요: ______________

저는 위의 내용을 전부 읽었고 질문에 대한 답도 다 들었습니다. 저는 정맥 조영술 실시에 동의합니다.

______________ ______________
환자/보호자 서명과 날짜 증인 서명과 날짜

저는 위의 내용을 읽었고 선택에 대해 논의했습니다. 저는 조영제 시술에 동의하지 않습니다. 저는 조영제 없이 검사하는 것이 적합하지 않거나 충분하지 않은 정보를 제공하는 결과를 가져올 수 있다는 것을 이해합니다.

______________ ______________
환자/보호자 서명과 날짜 증인 서명과 날짜

Consent ⑤ Consent for Contrast Material Injection 영문본 【1】

Hospital Name CONSENT FOR CONTRAST MATERIAL INJECTION	NAME CONSUMER NUMBER DATA OF BIRTH

You are having an exam requiring the injection of contrast material(x-ray dye). The contrast is given through a small catheter(IV) placed into a vein. The injection is necessary to facilitate the performance and interpretation of your exam. Without contrast, the exam may provide inadequate or less sufficient diagnostic information.

Contrast injections are given frequently and considered routine. Mild adverse reaction to the contrast occurs in about 1 in 250 to 1 in 500 patients. Mild reactions include sneezing, hives, scratchy throats, watery eyes, nausea, etc.

These symptoms are temporary and usually subside by themselves or with antihistamines.

Major reactions(drop in blood pressure, respiratory distress, cardiac arrest, loss of consciousness, kidney failure, etc.) occur in about 1 in 5,000 patients. Death has occurred in about 1 in 75,000 injections. Rarely, contrast may leak from the vein. This may cause severe tissue damage and may require surgery to attempt correction. Permanent scarring and/or nerve or muscle damage may also occur as a result of the leakage or surgery.

Please answer the following questions to assist us to provide the optimal care.

1. Age: ______________
2. Do you have any allergies(include medicinal, environmental, and food allergies)? YES NO
   If YES, please list:______________________________
3. Have you ever had a prior allergic reaction to contrast material(x-ray dye)? YES NO
   If YES, describe the type of reaction:______________________________
4. Do you have the following health problems/illnesses?

________ Asthma	________ Heart Problems	________ High Blood Pressure
________ Diabetes	________ Multiple Myeloma	________ Sickle Cell Disease
________ Pheochromocytoma	________ Kidney Disease	________ Polycythemia

   Other:______________________________
5. Are you pregnant? YES NO Are you breast-feeding YES NO
6. Please list your current medications:______________________________

I have read the above information and my questions have been answered. I agree to the administration of TV contrast material.

______________________________ ______________________________

Patient/Guardian Signature and Date Witness Signature and Date

I have read the above information and discussed the options. I do not wish to have IV contrast administration. I understand that, without the contrast, the exam may provide inadequate or insufficient diagnostic information.

______________________________ ______________________________

Patient/Guardian Signature and Date Witness Signature and Date

Consent ⑤ Consent for Contrast Material Injection (Radiology) 한글본 【2】

조영제 주사 실시동의서	이름 ______ 생년월일 ______

방사선과 기록

조영제 주사 실시자:____________장소:_______종류/크기:________위치:

정맥주사 종결자:___________장소:__________부위: 정상　　　카테터 무손상 네　　아니오
붉게 됨
침윤물

조영제 실시자: ____

양: ____ CC

방사선과 의사명: ____

혈청 크레아티닌 ________________날짜________________
(밀리그램/디시리터)　　　(날짜)

반응:	네/아니오	대답이 '네'인 경우 약부작용 대한 내용을 기록하세요.		
타입:	I	II	III	IV
치료법:	A	B	C	
조영제 혈관외 유출:	네/아니오	대답이 '네'인 경우 조영제 유출에 대한 내용을 기록하세요.		

의견: ____

____

____

____

____

____

Consent ⑤ Consent for Contrast Material Injection (Radiology) 영문본 【2】

CONSENT FOR CONTRAST MATERIAL INJECTION	NAME ______ Date of Birth ______

FOR RADIOLOGY DEPARTMENT USE ONLY

I.V. start by:__________at:__________Type/size:__________Location:

I.V. line D/C'd by:__________at:__________site: Normal Catheter Intact: YES NO
Redness
Infiltrate

Contrast injected by: __________

Amount: __________ cc's

Radiologist: __________

Serum Creatinine __________on__________
(mg/dl) (date)

Reaction:	YES/NO	IF YES, complete Adverse Drug Reaction Form.			
Type:	I		II	III	IV
Treatment:	A		B	C	
Contrast Extravasation:	YES/NO	IF YES, complete Contrast Media Extravasation Form.			

Comments: __________

단어 정리

☐ D/C'd(discontinued)	☐ 단절, 정지
☐ intact	☐ 무손상-, 완전한-
☐ redness	☐ 붉게 됨
☐ infiltrate	☐ 침윤물
☐ radiologist	☐ 방사선과 의사
☐ extravasation	☐ 혈관밖 유출, 유출
☐ adverse Drug Reaction	☐ 약에 대한 부작용

⑥ 환자 정보 요청 허가서(Consent for Release of Information)

□ 원칙

환자의 어떤 의료 정보도 환자 또는 법적 보호자의 허가 없이 요청할 수 없다. 환자가 진찰받는 데 다른 의료기관이나 그 외 장소에서 받은 모든 진찰에 대한 내용을 요청하게 된다. 이때 허가서를 작성하고 그 허가서를 다른 의료기관에 제시할 때에만 환자 정보를 요청하고 수렴할 수 있다. 허가서는 환자 또는 법적 보호자의 서명과 날짜가 반드시 명시되어야 한다.

□ 시행

환자의 의료기록을 요청하면 전자 문서일 때는 전송하는 방법으로 또 문서일 경우에는 팩스나 혹은 직접적 문서 전달 등의 방법으로 전달된다. 요청하는 허가서 작성 시 어떤 정보들이 기록되어야 하는지 살펴보자.

- 환자 이름
- 진료 자료를 요청할 의료기관 명칭
- 진료 자료를 받을 의료기관 명칭
- 요청하는 특정 자료 내용
- 환자 자신, 혹은 법적 보호자의 서명
  서명이 환자 자신이 아닐 경우에는 환자와의 관계를 명시한다.
  환자가 서명하지 않는 경우는 18살 이하인 경우, 18살 이상이지만 정신적 결함이 있을 경우 등이다.
- 서명 날짜: 1년 이상이 초과된 경우 대개 무효화된다.
- 요청서가 언제든지 파기될 수 있다는 내용 명시

□ 요청서 없이 진료 자료를 요청할 수 있는 경우

- 응급 상황일 경우
- 학교 내 양호시설에서 필요한 경우
- 정부에서 법적 조치를 위해 요구할 경우
- 통계자료일 경우

• 연구자료일 경우
• 법원 요청이 있을 경우 등

□ 구두 요청만으로도 가능한 경우
• 환자 본인이 직접 요청한 경우 신분을 확인하고 자료를 받을 수 있다.
• 환자가 의식이 있지만 응급한 경우 구두로 요청할 수 있다.

Consent ⑥ Consent for Release of Information 한글본 【1】

의료기관 이름

환자 정보 개방 요청서

날짜 ______________________

1. 저는 (의료기관 명)__________에게 (환자이름)__________의 의료기록 내용 중에 다음 정보를 개방해도 좋다는 것을 수락합니다.
   주소____
   입원기간 의료기록:
   입원날짜____
   퇴원날짜____
   병원 고유번호 #__________________________생년월일____________________

2. 개방을 원하는 정보
   【 】 의료기록지 복사본 【 】 퇴원기록지
   【 】 병력과 신체검사 결과 【 】 수술기록지
   【 】 그 외____

3. 정보를 개방할 대상(의료기관 또는 의료진이름)
   ____

4. 개방의 목적____

5. 이 허락서로 인정되어 이미 발생한 개방에 대한 것을 제외하고는 이 허가서는 언제든지 무효화될 수 있다는 것을 이해한다.

6. 특정 날짜, 사건, 조건

7. 기관, 고용인들, 사무직원, 담당 의사는 위의 정보 개방에 대해 특별히 명시되지 않는 한 법적 책임 혹은 의무가 없다.

서명__________________________________

(환자 혹은 환자 보호자)

____

(환자와의 관계)

____

(서명 날짜)

Consent ⑥ Consent for Release of Information 영문본 【1】

NAME OF FACILITY

CONSENT FOR RELEASE OF INFORMATION

DATE ________________________

1. I hereby authorize____________________(the Name of Institution) to release following information from the health record(s) of (Patient Name) ____________________________
Address____
Covering the period(s) of hospitalization from:
Date of Admission____
Date of Discharge____
Hospital #________________________________Birthdate_____________________________

2. Information to be released

【 】 Copy of(complete)health record(s) 【 】 Discharge Summary

【 】 History and Physical 【 】 Operative Report

【 】 Other____

3. Information is to be release to____

4. Purpose of disclosure____

5. I understand this consent can be revoked at any time except to the extent that disclosure made in good faith has already occurred in reliance on this consent.

6. Specification of the date, event, or condition upon which this consent expires.

7. The facility, its employees and officers and attending physician are released from legal responsibility or liability for the release of the above information to the extent indicated and authorized herein.

Signed____
(Patient or Representative)

____
(Relationship to Patient)

____
(Date of Signature)

환자 의료기록 개방 허락서

환자 이름: ______________________________ 생년월일: ______________

1. 저는 (의료기관 명)에 요청하며 권한을 부여해드립니다.
   - -에 정보를 개방해 주실 것을
   - -로부터 정보를 요청할 것을
2. 의료서비스 제공자/기관 ______________________________

   주소 ______________________________

   전화번호 ______________ 연락할 수 있는 사람 ______________
3. 개방 요청의 목적(해당되는 사항을 모두 표시하세요)
   - 이사
   - 건강보험에 필요
   - 다른 진료소 방문
   - 2차적 의견
   - 개인검토
   - 그 외(내용을 적어 주세요) ______________________________
4. 다음과 같은 기밀이 유지되어야 하는 건강정보가 개방될 것입니다. (한 가지만 선택하여 표시해 주세요)
   - 저는 기록, 보고서, 알코올 중독과 그에 관한 테스트 그리고/혹은 마약중독과 그 치료 내력, 성병 그리고/혹은 심리적 혹은 정신과적 치료를 포함하는 모든 의료기록의 개방을 원합니다.
   - 저는 다음 열거하는 내용을 제외한 나머지 정보만 개방하기를 요청합니다.(개방을 원하지 않는 정보를 열거하십시오) ______________________________

     ____

     ____
   - 저는 다음 열거한 치료나 증세에 대한 정보를 제외한 나머지 정보의 개방을 요청합니다.

     ____
   - 저는 ________부터 _______까지(기간)의 모든 의료기록의 개방을 요청합니다.
5. 이 권한 부여는 서명한 날로부터 1년이 되면 자동적으로 무효화됩니다. 저는 이미 저의 요청으로 개방이 일어날 경우를 제외하고는 서면으로 이 요청을 언제든지 취소할 수 있다는 것을 인정합니다.

______________________________ ______________

환자의 서명/환자 대리인/법적 보호자 날짜

______________________________ ______________

증인 날짜

정보 수취자/기관: 법으로 기밀성이 유지되어 있는 이 정보가 본인 혹은 기관에 개방되었습니다. 법적으로 이 정보를 특정한 서면상의 허락 없이는 어디에도 개방할 수 없도록 제한하고 있음을 알려드립니다.

CONSENT FOR RELEASE OF MEDICAL INFORMATION

Patient Name: ______________________________ DOB: ______________

1. I hereby request and authorize (name of Medical facility) to:
   - Release Information TO
   - Obtain Information FROM

2. Name of Provider/Facility ______________________________
   Address ______________________________
   Telephone ______________ Contact Person ______________

3. The PURPOSE of this release is: (check all that apply)
   - Moving
   - Insurance Purpose
   - Transferring Care
   - Second Opinion
   - Personal Review
   - Other (please specify) ______________________________

4. The FOLLOWING Protected Health Information (PHI) may be released: (please check one)
   - I consent to the release of all medical records including records, reports or tests concerning alcoholism and/or drug abuse or treatment information, sexually transmitted disease related and/or psychological or psychiatric treatment. I also understand that the release of information related to the diagnosis or treatment of HIV requires an additional authorization.
   - I consent to the release of all medical records with the following exceptions. (Specifically describe the information you do not wish to have released) ______________________________
     ____
     ____
   - I consent to the release of all medical records relating to the following treatment or condition:
     ____
   - I consent to the release of all medical records from __________ to __________.

5. This authorization will automatically expire within one year from the date of signature.
   I understand that I have the right to revoke this authorization in writing at any time, except where information has already been released in response to this authorization.

______________________________ ______________

Signature of Patient/Representative/or Legal Guardian Date

______________________________ ______________

Witness Date

NOTICE TO RECIPIENT OF RECORDS: This information has been disclosed to you from confidential records that are protected by law. This law prohibits you from making any future disclosures of this information without specific written authorization of the person to whom it pertains.

V. 안내문

안내문 ① 건강검진프로그램

건강검진프로그램

■ 목적

• 건강검진은 발병 이전에 치료를 요하는 건강 문제들을 확인할 수 있게 하여 병의 예방 및 치료에 드는 비용을 줄일 수 있게 할 것입니다. 예방이 병의 발병을 피하고 비용을 낮출 수 있는 최상의 방법입니다. 종합건강검진은 각 분야의 검사와 상담을 의미하며 더 나아가서 전문의와의 개인상담 기회를 제공합니다.

■ 준비

• 검진 12시간 전에는 금식하셔야 하며 물만 마실 수 있습니다. 검사 당일에는 평상시 의사에게 간단한 치료를 받을 때처럼, 편안한 옷차림으로 오십시오.

■ 절차

• 도착하시면 간호사가 혈액 샘플을 채취할 것입니다.

• 검사 시, 소변 샘플도 요구됩니다.

• 의사가 과거, 현재 상태, 백신접종 여부, 사전검사, 테스트 결과 등의 병력에 대해 질문할 것입니다. 환자분이 궁금하거나, 통증을 느끼는 건강 문제에 대해 상담할 수 있는 기회가 될 것입니다(상담은 내과 전문의에 의해서 기본 검진과 함께 시행됩니다).

• 검진 시, 이런 증상에 대해 논의할 시간을 충분히 가지실 수 있습니다.

• 의사가 운동 습관, 일반 식사 습관, 흡연, 수면, 스트레스 지수, 가족 및 직장 생활을 포함한 생활 습관에 대해 질문할 것입니다.

• 전체적인 건강검진은 몸무게, 신장, 혈압, 심장, 폐, 위, 시력, 청력, 후비강, 갑상선, 반사작용 등을 포함할 것입니다.

• 원하시는 분에 한해, 남성은 전립선 검사를, 여성은 자궁 검사를 받으실 수 있습니다.

■ 검사결과

• 검사가 완료되면 건강에 대한 총체적인 상황을 확인하실 수 있습니다. 현재 건강에 대한 개인적, 실제적 정보를 제시하여 미래 건강을 위한 계획을 세울 수 있습니다.

• 검사결과는 검진자의 건강목표, 미래 건강 예상, 건강에 도움이 되는 생활 습관 등을 즉각적으로 시행할 수 있도록 제시하여 줄 수 있습니다.

뒷장으로 넘겨주십시오.

건강검진프로그램

1. 기본 건강검진프로그램

1) 신장, 체중, 혈압, 체성분

2) 혈액검사: 각종 혈액검사 70가지

3) 체지방검사: 체지방 분석

4) 소변검사: 요단백, 요당, 요잠혈, 빌리루빈, 요비중, 요pH

5) 대변검사: 잠혈

6) 시력검사: 안압 검사

7) 청력검사: 좌, 우(1000, 2000, 4000, 8000 주파수)

2. 장기별 정밀진단과 임상적 의의

1) 심장검사: 심근경색, 협심증, 부정맥 등 심장별 관련 질환 정밀 검사－심전도 검사

2) 소화기 검사: 소화기계통에 호발하는 위암, 간암, 췌장암, 대장암 등의 정밀진단－위장 조영 촬영, 위내시경 검사

3) 흉부검사: 폐결핵, 폐렴, 폐암 등의 정밀진단－흉부 X선 촬영(정명/측면), 폐기능 검사

4) 뇌정밀검사: 뇌졸중(중풍)을 비롯한 뇌혈관 기형, 뇌암, 파킨슨병 등 뇌질환에 대한 정밀진단－뇌혈관검사(MRA), 인슐린 분비능력 검사(C-peptide), 경동맥 초음파

5) 척추검사: 디스크 등 척추관련 질환 조기발견－MRI(요추, 경추), 요추 X선 촬영, 경추 X선 촬영

6) 여성정밀: 난소종양, 자궁근종, 골다공증, 유방암, 갑상선질환 등 여성에게 흔히 발생하는 질환에 대한 진단－골밀도검사, 유방암검사, 자궁암검사, 여성호르몬검사, 골반초음파, 갑상선 동위원소 촬영

7) 구강검사: 우식증, 결손치, 치주염 검사

안내문 ① 건강검진프로그램 【영문번역】

건강검진프로그램
Health Screening Programs

■ 목적(Purpose)

• 건강검진은 발병 이전에 치료를 요하는 건강 문제들을 확인할 수 있게 하여 병의 예방 및 치료에 드는 비용을 줄일 수 있게 할 것입니다. 예방이 병의 발병을 피하고 비용을 낮출 수 있는 최상의 방법입니다. 종합건강검진은 각 분야의 검사와 상담을 의미하며 더 나아가서 전문의와의 개인상담 기회를 제공합니다.
Your health exam will bring up your health issues that need special attention, taking care of them now could avoid more costly treatment in future. Prevention is the best way to keep you avoids any medical problems and lowers your cost. The comprehensive physical examination is equal parts examination and consultation, and provides the opportunity for an extended, one-on-one Specialist doctor visit.

■ 준비(Preparation)

• 검진 12시간 전에는 금식하셔야 하며 물만 마실 수 있습니다. 검사 당일에는 평상시 의사에게 간단한 치료를 받을 때처럼, 편안한 옷차림으로 오십시오.
12 hours before the exam you will fast in preparation and drink only the plain water. The day of the exam you should dress in comfortable clothing, as you would for a physical exam with your own doctor.

■ 절차(Procedure)

• 도착하시면 간호사가 혈액 샘플을 채취할 것입니다.
On your arrival, a nurse will draw samples for the laboratory blood tests.

• 검사 시, 소변 샘플도 요구됩니다.
A urine sample will also be requested sometime during your visit.

• 의사가 과거, 현재 상태, 백신접종 여부, 사전검사, 테스트 결과 등의 병력에 대해 질문할 것입니다. 환자분이 궁금하거나, 통증을 느끼는 건강 문제에 대해 상담할 수 있는 기회가 될 것입니다(상담은 내과 전문의에 의해서 기본 검진과 함께 시행됩니다).
The physician will interview you (carried out by our specialist of internal medicine upon completion of your full check up program) about your health history, including past and current conditions, vaccines, previous screenings and test results. This is an excellent opportunity to bring up any and all health questions or issues that you are curious about, or that have been bothering you.

• 검진 시, 이런 증상에 대해 논의할 시간을 충분히 가지실 수 있습니다.
You'll have plenty of time to talk about them during your visit.

• 의사가 운동 습관, 일반 식사 습관, 흡연, 수면, 스트레스 지수, 가족 및 직장 생활을 포함한 생활 습관에 대해 질문할 것입니다.
The physician will also ask you about your lifestyle including exercise habits, general diet, smoking habits, sleeping habits, stress level, and family and work life.

• 전체적인 건강검진은 몸무게, 신장, 혈압, 심장, 폐, 위, 시력, 청력, 후비강, 갑상선, 반사작용 등을 포함할 것입니다.
The extremely thorough physical examination will include checks of your weight, height, blood pressure, heart, lungs, abdomen, vision, ears, throat, thyroid, reflexes.

• 원하시는 분에 한해, 남성은 전립선 검사를, 여성은 자궁 검사를 받으실 수 있습니다.
Men will receive a prostate exam, and women will receive a pelvic exam if they request it at the time they schedule their appointment.

■ 검사결과(What it shows)

• 검사가 완료되면 건강에 대한 총체적인 상황을 확인하실 수 있습니다. 현재 건강에 대한 개인적, 실제적 정보를 제시하여 미래 건강을 위한 계획을 세울 수 있습니다.
When it is done, you will have a complete picture of your health. It will give you a very personal and practical information for now and the direction for the future.

• 검사결과는 검진자의 건강목표, 미래 건강 예상, 건강에 도움이 되는 생활 습관 등을 즉각적으로 시행할 수 있도록 제시하여 줄 수 있습니다.
They also will take into account your unique goals, perspective and lifestyle which will work in a unique way for you so that you can put to use immediately.

1. 기본 건강검진 프로그램(Basic Health Screening Program)

1) 신장, 체중, 혈압, 체성분
Height, Weight, Blood pressure

2) 혈액검사: 각종 혈액검사 70가지
Complete blood test: 70types of blood tests

3) 체지방검사: 체지방 분석
Body composition, body fat analysis

4) 소변검사: 요단백, 요당, 요잠혈, 빌리루빈, 요비중, 요pH
Urine test: urine protein, urine sugar, urine occult blood, bilirubin, urinometry, urine pH

5) 대변검사: 잠혈
Stool test: fecal occult blood

6) 시력검사: 안압 검사
Eye exam: tonometry (eye pressure test)

7) 청력검사: 좌, 우(1000, 2000, 4000, 8000 주파수)
Hearing test: left and right hearing frequency test(1000, 2000, 4000, 8000)

2. 장기별 정밀진단과 임상적 의의(Extensive Health Exams and Tests)

1) 심장검사: 심근경색, 협심증, 부정맥 등 심장별 관련 질환 정밀 검사－심전도 검사
Cardiovascular Exam: mayocardial infarction, angina, arrhythmia and so on
－ECG(electrocardiogram)

2) 소화기 검사: 소화기계통에 호발하는 위암, 간암, 췌장암, 대장암 등의 정밀진단－위장 조영 촬영, 위내시경 검사
Gastoenterologic Exam:
gastric cancer, liver cancer, pancreas cancer, colon cancer－UGI(UpperGastrointestinography), gastro endoscopy

3) 흉부검사: 폐결핵, 폐렴, 폐암 등의 정밀진단－흉부 X선 촬영(정명/측면), 폐기능 검사
Chest Exam: tuberculosis, pneumonia, lung cancer
－Chest X-ray(front/side), PFT(pulmonary function test)

4) 뇌정밀검사: 뇌졸중(중풍)을 비롯한 뇌혈관 기형, 뇌암, 파킨슨병 등 뇌질환에 대한 정밀진단－뇌혈관검사(MRA), 인슐린 분비능력 검사(C-peptide), 경동맥 초음파
Brain Scan: cerebrovascula deformity, brain cancer, Parkinson's disease, stroke
－cerebrovascular examination (Magnetic Resonance Angiography, MRA), Insulin secretion capacity test (C-peptide), carotid ultrasound test

5) 척추검사: 디스크 등 척추관련 질환 조기 발견－MRI(요추, 경추), 요추 X선 촬영, 경추 X선 촬영
Spinal Exam: an early detection of spinal disease, herniated disk
－MRI (lumbar, cervical), lumbar X-ray, cervical X-ray]

6) 여성정밀: 난소종양, 자궁근종, 골다공증, 유방암, 갑상선질환 등 여성에게 흔히 발생하는 질환에 대한 진단－골밀도검사, 유방암검사, 자궁암검사, 여성호르몬검사, 골반초음파, 갑상선 동위원소 촬영
Comprehensive women's health check-ups: ovarian tumor, fibroid, osteoporosis, thyroiditis
－bone density test, cancer screening(breast, cervical, uterine and ovary), hormone test, pelvic ultrasound exam, isotope thyroid scan

7) 구강검사: 우식증, 결손치, 치주염검사
Dental Exam: dental caries, defective teeth, periodontitis

안내문 ② 위내시경 검사

■ 검사 전 준비사항

• 위내시경 검사는 환자의 식도, 위, 십이지장을 내시경을 이용해 검사하는 과정입니다.
• 검사를 통해 환자의 여러 가지 증세—삼키기 힘든 증상, 메스꺼움, 구토, 역류, 출혈, 소화불량, 복통 혹은 속쓰림 등의 증상—의 원인을 발견하기 위한 과정입니다.
• 철저하고 안전한 위내시경을 실시하기 위해 위와 십이지장을 비워야만 합니다.
• 적어도 8시간 이상 음식을 먹거나 물을 마시면 안 됩니다.
• 저녁은 6시경 죽이나 미음으로 드시고 물은 자정까지만 드십시오.
• 자정 이후부터는 아무것도 드시지 마십시오.
• 검사 당일 아침에 양치질을 깨끗이 하고 화장을 하거나 립스틱을 바르지 마시고 오십시오.

■ 검사 전 주의사항

• 당뇨 환자 중 인슐린을 주사하는 분은 당일 절반 용량만 주사하고 오십시오.
• 아스피린, 코마딘과 같은 항응고제를 복용하는 경우, 약 복용 여부를 담당 진료의사와 미리 상의 후 오셔야 합니다.
• 현재 고혈압 약을 복용하고 계시다면, 오전 5시에 혈압약을 복용하고 오십시오.
• 검사 당일 반드시 보호자와 함께 오시고 사고의 위험이 있으므로 시술 후 운전하시면 안 됩니다.
• 검사 과정과 합병증에 대한 내용이 포함된 검사 승낙서에 서명합니다.

■ 검사과정

• 검사 전 활력 징후(체온, 혈압, 맥박, 호흡 등)를 측정할 것입니다.
• 약에 대한 알레르기 반응이 있으신 분은 간호사에게 말씀해 주십시오.
• 검사 전 틀니가 있으신 분은 미리 틀니를 제거하세요.
• 입에 마우스피스를 물어야 합니다.
• 먼저 가늘고, 부드러운 비경 내시경을 삽입합니다.
• 시술 직전에 의사는 목을 마취시키기 위해 부분 마취약을 주고, 진통제를 줄 것입니다.
• 검사 중 편안하게 잠을 주무시도록 안정제를 검사 시작 직전에 정맥주사로 주입합니다.
• 비경 내시경을 코를 통하여 목, 식도, 위, 십이지장으로 서서히 삽입하면서 조직의 이상 유무를 확인합니다.
• 필요에 따라 검사 및 치료목적으로 조직검사를 시행하게 됩니다.
• 검사 중 의사는 내시경 기구를 통해 공기를 주입할 것입니다; 이렇게 하여 내부의 접힌 부분을 열고 내부 벽을 쉽게 관찰할 수 있게 해줍니다.
• 주입으로 인한 복부 불편감이 있을 수 있으며 구역질 반응이 있을 수 있습니다.
• 이때 온몸에 힘을 빼고 침은 삼키지 말고 옆으로 흘러내리도록 하고 호흡은 입으로 들이쉬고 내쉬는 심호흡을 하면서 참아야 합니다.
• 검사 중 자세는 다음과 같이 왼편으로 누워 다리를 약간 구부린 상태로 10~15분 정도 검사를 받게 됩니다.

■ 검사 후 주의사항

• 검사 종료 시 회복실로 이동한 후 깨어날 때까지 간호사가 관찰할 것입니다.
• 의료진의 별다른 지시가 없으면 바로 식사 가능합니다. 단, 조직 검사를 한 경우에는 출혈의 위험이 있으므로 1시간가량 후에 식사를 하십시오.

• 조직 검사 시행 후 다음과 같은 증상이 있을 경우 바로 병원에 연락하십시오. - 출혈이 있는 경우 - 흑색 변을 보거나 - 피를 토하거나 - 심하게 어지럽고 - 맥박이 빨라지거나 - 식은땀이 나며 - 심한 복부 통증이 있을 경우
■ 검사결과 상담
• 깨어나신 후 담당 의사로부터 사전 상담하실 수 있습니다. • 그러나 자세한 검사결과는 담당 의사 선생님께 보내질 것입니다. • 조직 검사결과는 다음 약속 때 받아 보실 수 있습니다. • 귀가하시기 전에 다음 약속을 하고 가십시오.

안내문 ② 위내시경 검사 【영문번역】

■ 검사 전 준비사항(Preparation for the Procedure)

• 위내시경 검사는 환자의 식도, 위, 십이지장을 내시경을 이용해 검사하는 과정입니다.
Upper Gastrointestinal Endoscopy is the procedure which enables to look inside esophagus, stomach, and duodenums.

• 검사를 통해 환자의 여러 가지 증세—삼키기 힘든 증상, 메쓰거움, 구토, 역류, 출혈, 소화불량, 복통 혹은 속쓰림 등의 증상—의 원인을 발견하기 위한 과정입니다.
The procedure is used to discover the reason for swallowing difficulties, nausea, vomiting, reflux, bleeding, indigestion, abdominal pain, or heartburn.

• 철저하고 안전한 위내시경을 실시하기 위해 위와 십이지장을 비워야만 합니다.
Your stomach and duodenum must be empty for the procedure to be thorough and safe.

• 적어도 8시간 이상 음식을 먹거나 물을 마시면 안 됩니다.
So you will not be able to eat or drink anything for at least 8 hours.

• 저녁은 6시경 죽이나 미음으로 드시고 물은 자정까지만 드십시오.
Please have liquid meal for your dinner at 6 P.M. and drink water only until midnight.

• 자정 이후부터는 아무것도 드시지 마십시오.
Completely stop eating and drinking from midnight.

• 검사 당일 아침에 양치질을 깨끗이 하고 화장을 하거나 립스틱을 바르지 마시고 오십시오.
On the day of your exam, brush your teeth and avoid to wear any make up or lip stick.

■ 검사 전 주의사항(Before the Procedure)

• 당뇨 환자 중 인슐린을 주사하는 분은 당일 절반 용량만 주사하고 오십시오.
If you are diabetic and taking insulin injection, you can inject only half dose before you admit to the hospital for the procedure.

• 아스피린, 코마딘과 같은 항응고제를 복용하는 경우, 약 복용 여부를 담당 진료의사와 미리 상의 후 오셔야 합니다.
If you are currently taking anticoagulant drug, such as Coumadin or aspirin, you should discuss with your physician beforehand.

• 현재 고혈압 약을 복용하고 계시다면, 오전 5시에 혈압약을 복용하고 오십시오.
If you are currently taking medicine for the high blood pressure, take medicine at 5 in the morning.

• 검사 당일 반드시 보호자와 함께 오시고 사고의 위험이 있으므로 시술 후 운전하시면 안 됩니다.
You must arrange for someone to take you home. You will not be allowed to drive because of the sedatives.

• 검사 과정과 합병증에 대한 내용이 포함된 검사 승낙서에 서명합니다.
You will be asked to sign a consent form authorizing the physician to perform the procedure.

■ 검사과정(Procedure)

• 검사 전 활력 징후(체온, 혈압, 맥박, 호흡 등)를 측정할 것입니다.
The nurse will take your temperature, blood pressure, pulse and respiration rate.

• 약에 대한 알레르기 반응이 있으신 분은 간호사에게 말씀해 주십시오.
Please let the nurse know if you are allergic to any medication.

• 검사 전 틀니가 있으신 분은 미리 틀니를 제거하세요.
You must remove your dentures before the procedure.

• 입에 마우스피스를 물어야 합니다.
A mouthpiece will be placed in your mouth.

• 먼저 가늘고, 부드러운 비경 내시경을 삽입합니다.
For the procedure you will swallow a narrow, flexible tube called an endoscope.

• 시술 직전에 의사는 목을 마취시키기 위해 부분 마취약을 주고, 진통제를 줄 것입니다.
Right before the procedure, a local anesthetic (pain-relieving medication) may be applied at the back of your throat. numbing agent and you will receive pain medicine.

• 검사 중 편안하게 잠을 주무시도록 안정제를 검사시작 직전에 정맥주사로 주입합니다.
A sedative will be given intravenously (in your vein) that will make you relaxed and drowsy.

• 비경 내시경을 코를 통하여 목, 식도, 위, 십이지장으로 서서히 삽입하면서 조직의 이상 유무를 확인합니다.
The doctor will insert the endoscope into your mouth, through your esophagus (the "food pipe" leading from your mouth into your stomach) and into your stomach.
The physician can see any abnormalities while the endoscope slide down through esophagus, stomach, and duodenum.

• 필요에 따라 검사 및 치료목적으로 조직검사를 시행하게 됩니다.
Biopsy will be done for the lab test and appropriate treatment, when it is needed.

• 검사 중 의사는 내시경 기구를 통해 공기를 주입할 것입니다; 이렇게 하여 내부의 접힌 부분을 열고 내부 벽을 쉽게 관찰할 수 있게 해 줍니다.
The physician will place air in the stomach through the scope; this opens the folds of stomach and makes it easier for the physician to examine the lining of these organs.

• 주입으로 인한 복부 불편감이 있을 수 있으며 구역질반응이 있을 수 있습니다.
You might feel stomach bloating, or/and nausea due to place the air inside.

• 이때 온몸에 힘을 빼고 침은 삼키지 말고 옆으로 흘러내리도록 하고 호흡은 입으로 들이쉬고 내쉬는 심호흡을 하면서 참아야 합니다.

Please relax and do not swallow saliva, rather you can let the saliva flowing to the side. Take a deep breath through your mouth and try to be patient as much as possible.

• 검사 중 자세는 다음과 같이 왼편으로 누워 다리를 약간 구부린 상태로 10~15분 정도 검사를 받게 됩니다.
You will lie on your left side with your legs bend during the procedure. Most procedures will take 10 to 15 minutes.

■ 검사 후 주의사항(After the Procedure)

• 검사 종료 시 회복실로 이동한 후 깨어날 때까지 간호사가 관찰할 것입니다.
When all the procedure is over, you will be transferred to the recovery room and closely observed by the nurse until you are awake.

• 의료진의 별다른 지시가 없으면 바로 식사 가능합니다. 단, 조직 검사를 한 경우에는 출혈의 위험이 있으므로 1시간가량 후에 식사를 하십시오.
You can have a meal unless otherwise instructed. However, if you had biopsy, you can have a meal 1 hour after the procedure since there might be a chance of bleeding.

• 조직 검사 시행 후 다음과 같은 증상이 있을 경우 바로 병원에 연락하십시오
- 출혈이 있는 경우
- 흑색 변을 보거나
- 피를 토하거나
- 심하게 어지럽고
- 맥박이 빨라지거나
- 식은땀이 나며
- 심한 복부 통증이 있을 경우

Please contact us as quick as possible if you have following symptoms after the procedure.
- bleeding
- dark stool
- vomit blood
- severe drowsiness
- palpitation
- cold sweating
- severe stomache

■ 검사결과 상담(Discussion for the Result)

• 깨어나신 후 담당 의사로부터 사전 상담하실 수 있습니다.
Preliminary findings will be discussed with your doctor after you awake.

• 그러나 자세한 검사결과는 담당 의사 선생님께 보내질 것입니다.
A full report will be sent to your doctor.
• 조직 검사결과는 다음 약속 때 받아 보실 수 있습니다.
Biopsy results will be available at your next appointment.

• 귀가하시기 전에 다음 약속을 하고 가십시오.
Please make a follow up appointment before you leave.

안내문 ③ 양전자방출단층촬영(PET: Positron Emission Tomography), PET-CT

■ 개요 및 원리
• PET-CT 검사는 핵의학 영상을 통한 진단법입니다. • 핵의학은 의학적 영상진단법 중의 하나로 소량의 방사선 물질을 사용하여 각종 질병－암, 심장병, 소화기계, 비뇨기계, 신경계 질환들을 초기에 발견하고 진단하여 효과적인 치료 방법들을 결정할 수 있게 됩니다. • 영상을 통해 중요한 인체 기능, 즉 혈액 순환, 산소 소비 그리고 당 대사 작용 등을 측정하여 의사가 기관과 조직의 기능이 어떤지를 평가할 수 있습니다. • PET-CT 전에, 환자는 방사선 반응 포도당을 정맥주사로 투여받게 됩니다. • 악성 종양(암세포)조직은 양성 및 정상조직과 다르게 대사 작용이 높고, 포도당과 빠르게 합성합니다. • 전신 PET-CT 검사를 통해 발견되는 포도당의 비정상적 분포 위치에 대한 정보에 의해 의사들은 암의 발생 위치, 암의 전이 상태 등을 효과적으로 진단할 수 있습니다.
■ 임상적 의의
• 폐암, 유방암, 뇌종양, 간암, 식도암, 림프육종, 뼈에 생긴 암, 난소암, 자궁암 등, 간질, 치매, 뇌혈관 질환, 심근 경색, 각종 관상동맥질환
■ 방사성의약품
• 18F-FDG
■ 검사 전 준비
• 검사를 위해서 8～12시간 전부터 금식하여야 합니다. • 물(생수)은 가능한 많이 드시는 것이 좋습니다. • 오렌지 주스, 커피, 콜라, 홍차, 녹차 등 당분이 함유된 물을 드시면 절대 안 됩니다. • 검사 시작 전에 혈당 검사를 위하여 채혈을 진행하게 되며 혈당이 너무 높거나 낮은 경우에는 검사가 취소 또는 연기될 수 있습니다. • 임산부나 임신이 예상되는 분은 검사 전에 담당자에게 반드시 알려 주십시오. • PET- CT검사 시 조영제를 사용하게 되며, 조영제에 대한 부작용이 있으신 분은 검사 전에 미리 말씀해 주십시오.
■ 검사과정
• 검사를 위해서 먼저 이뇨제를 복용하고 키, 몸무게와 혈당을 측정하게 됩니다. • 검사를 위한 방사성의약품을 정맥주사하고, 대기실에 1시간 정도 계신 후 검사를 합니다. • 검사는 40～60분 정도 소요되며 편안하게 검사대에 누워 계시면 됩니다. • 검사대가 스캐너 안쪽으로 미끄러지듯 이동할 것입니다. • 검사 중에는 움직이지 않는 것이 중요합니다.
■ 검사 후 유의사항
• 검사 후 물을 많이 섭취하여 소변을 자주 보시면 방사성 의약품을 몸 밖으로 빨리 배출하는 데 도움이 됩니다.
■ 검사결과
• 검사결과는 영상학과 의사 선생님이 확인하고 환자분의 주치의에게 보고하실 것입니다. 다음 예약된 진료일에 주치의 선생님께 확인하면 됩니다.

안내문 ③ 양전자방출단층촬영(PET: Positron Emission Tomography), PET-CT 【영문번역】

■ 개요 및 원리(What is PET-CT?)

• PET-CT 검사는 핵의학 영상을 통한 진단법입니다.
PET-CT is a type of nuclear medicine imaging.

• 핵의학은 의학적 영상진단법 중의 하나로 소량의 방사선 물질을 사용하여 각종 질병－암, 심장병, 소화기계, 비뇨기계, 신경계 질환들을 초기에 발견하고 진단하여 효과적인 치료 방법들을 결정할 수 있게 됩니다.
Nuclear Medicine is a branch of medical imaging that uses small amounts of radioactive material to diagnose at the early stage and determine the effective treatments for a variety of diseases including cancers, heart diseases and gastrointestinal, endocrinal, neurological disorders.

• 영상을 통해 중요한 인체 기능, 즉 혈액 순환, 산소 소비 그리고 당 대사 작용 등을 측정하여 의사가 기관과 조직의 기능이 어떤지를 평가할 수 있습니다.
A PET scan measures important body functions, such as blood flow, oxygen use and sugar metabolism to help doctors evaluate how well organs and tissues are functioning.

• PET-CT 전에, 환자는 방사선 반응 포도당을 정맥주사로 투여받게 됩니다.
Before a PET-CT scan, the patient receives an intravenous injection of radioactive glucose.

• 악성 종양(암세포)조직은 양성 및 정상조직과 다르게 대사 작용이 높고, 포도당과 빠르게 합성합니다.
Many cancer cells are highly metabolic and rapidly synthesize the radioactive glucose which is different from normal tissue.

• 전신 PET-CT 검사를 통해 발견되는 포도당의 비정상적 분포 위치에 대한 정보에 의해 의사들은 암의 발생 위치, 암의 전이 상태 등을 효과적으로 진단할 수 있습니다.
Information regarding the location of abnormal levels of radioactive glucose obtained from the whole-body PET-CT scan helps physicians effectively pinpoint the source of cancer and detect whether cancer is isolated to one specific area or has spread to other organs.

■ 임상적 의의(Clinical Purpose)

• 폐암, 유방암, 뇌종양, 간암, 식도암, 림프육종, 뼈에 생긴 암, 난소암, 자궁암 등, 간질, 치매, 뇌혈관 질환, 심근 경색, 각종 관상동맥질환
Lung cancer, cerebral tumor, liver cancer, esophageal cancer, lymphosarcoma, bone cancer, ovarian cancer, uterine cancer etc., epilepsy, dimentia, cerebrovascular disease, myocardial infarction, various coronary artery disease

■ 방사성의약품(Radioactive Substance)

• 18F-FDG

■ 검사 전 준비(Preparation for the Procedure)

• 검사를 위해서 8～12시간 전부터 금식하여야 합니다.
You should fast for 8～12 hours before the procedure.

• 물(생수)은 가능한 많이 드시는 것이 좋습니다.
Patient should be well hydrated. Drink plenty of water. 500~1000 cc water is recommended.

• 오렌지 주스, 커피, 콜라, 홍차, 녹차 등 당분이 함유된 물을 드시면 절대 안 됩니다.
Please avoid any sugar-contained drink including orange juice, coffee, coke, tea or green tea.

• 검사 시작 전에 혈당 검사를 위하여 채혈을 진행하게 되며 혈당이 너무 높거나 낮은 경우에는 검사가 취소 또는 연기될 수 있습니다.
Before the exam, nurse will perform a finger-stick to test your glucose(sugar) level. If your glucose level is too high or too low, exam might be canceled or delayed.

• 임산부나 임신이 예상되는 분은 검사 전에 담당자에게 반드시 알려 주십시오.
You should inform to any imaging staff, if you are currently pregnant or eligible to be pregnant.

• PET-CT검사 시 조영제를 사용하게 되며, 조영제에 대한 부작용이 있으신 분은 검사 전에 미리 말씀해 주십시오.
Nurse will give you an injection of contrast agent for the procedure and you should notify us if you are allergic to this substance.

■ 검사과정(Procedure)

• 검사를 위해서 먼저 이뇨제를 복용하고 키, 몸무게와 혈당을 측정하게 됩니다.
Nurse will give you diuretics and check your height, weight and glucose level.

• 검사를 위한 방사성의약품을 정맥주사하고, 대기실에 1시간 정도 계신 후 검사를 합니다.
You will be injected radioactive substance through the IV line in your vein.
After the injection, you must wait for approximately 1 hour at the waiting room before the scanning can begin.

• 검사는 40~60분 정도 소요되며 편안하게 검사대에 누워 계시면 됩니다.
You will lie on your back on a scan table and be made as comfortable as possible.
The whole procedure will take approximately 40~60 minutes.

• 검사대가 스캐너 안쪽으로 미끄러지듯 이동할 것입니다.
The table will slide slowly into the middle of the scanner.

• 검사 중에는 움직이지 않는 것이 중요합니다.
It is important that you remain still throughout the scan.

■ 검사 후 유의사항(After the Procedure)

• 검사 후 물을 많이 섭취하여 소변을 자주 보시면 방사성 의약품을 몸 밖으로 빨리 배출하는 데 도움이 됩니다.
After the procedure, drink water as much as you can, so nuclear medicine can be quickly flush out from your system.

■ 검사결과(Result of Procedure)

• 검사결과는 영상학과 의사 선생님이 확인하고 환자분의 주치의에게 보고하실 것입니다. 다음 예약된 진료일에 주치의 선생님께 확인하면 됩니다.
The radiologist will interpret the scan and prepare a report for your doctor.
You can discuss about the result with your physician at your next appointment.

VI. 의료 서류에 쓰이는 용어들

1. 신체부위의 명칭(body parts and components)
(internal anatomy, external anatomy, body fluids, body substances)

	신체부위(Body part & component)	어원	의미
A	abdomen	lapar(o)-	복부
	aorta	aort(o)-	대동맥
	arm	brachi(o)-	팔
	armpit	-	겨드랑이
	artery	arteri(o)-	동맥
B	back	-	등
	big toe	-	엄지발가락
	bladder	cyst(o)-	방광
	blood	haemat-, hemat- (haem-, hem-)	혈액
	blood clot	thromb(o)-	혈전
	blood vessel	angi(o)-	혈관
	body	somat-, som-	신체
	bone	oste(o)-	뼈, 골
	bone marrow, marrow	myel(o)-	골수
	brain	encephal(o)-	뇌
	breast	mast(o)-	유방
C	chest	steth(o)-	가슴
	cheek	-	뺨
E	ear	ot(o)-	귀
	eggs, ova	oo-	난자
	eye	ophthalm(o)-	눈
	eyelid	blephar(o)-	눈꺼풀
F	face	prosop(o)-	얼굴
	fallopian tubes	salping(o)-	나팔관
	fat, fatty tissue	lip(o)-	지방 세포
	finger	dactyl(o)-	손가락
	forehead	-	이마
G	gallbladder	cholecyst(o)-	쓸개
	genitals, sexually undifferentiated	gon(o)-, phall(o)-	생식기
	gland	aden(o)-	선, 샘
	glanspenis or clitoridis	balan(o)-	귀두, 음핵

	신체부위(Body part & component)	어원	의미
G	gums	-	잇몸
H	hair	trich(o)-	모발
	hand	cheir(o)-, chir(o)-	손
	head	cephal(o)-	머리
	heart	cardi(o)-	심장
	hip, hip-joint	-	엉덩이(둔부), 고관절
	horn	cerat(o)-	촉각
I	intestine	enter(o)-	장(대장, 소장)
J	jaw	gnath(o)-	턱
K	kidney	nephr(o)-	신장
	knee	gon-	무릎
L	lip	cheil(o)-, chil(o)-	입술
	liver	hepat(o)- (hepatic-)	간
	loins, pubic region	episi(o)-	요부
	lungs	pneumon-	폐
M	marrow, bone marrow	myel(o)-	골수
	mind	psych-	마음
	mouth	stomat(o)-	입
	muscle	my(o)-	근육
N	nail	onych(o)-	손톱
	navel	omphal(o)-	배꼽
	neck	trachel(o)-	목
	nerve; the nervous system	neur(o)-	신경, 신경계
	nipple, teat	thele-	유두
	nose	rhin(o)-	코
O	ovary	oophor(o)-	난소
P	pelvis	pyel(o)-	골반
	penis	pe(o)-	음경
	pupil (of the eye)	cor-, core-, coro-	눈동자
R	rib	pleur(o)-	갈비뼈
	rib cage	thorac(i)-, thorac(o)-	흉곽
S	shoulder	om(o)-	어깨
	sinus	-	공동
	skin	dermat(o)- (derm-)	피부
	skull	crani(o)-	두개골
	stomach	gastr(o)-	위

	신체부위(Body part & component)	어원	의미
T	testis	orchi(o)-, orchid(o)-	고환
	throat (upper throat cavity)	pharyng(o)-	목
	throat (lower throat cavity/voice box])	laryng(o)-	목청
	thumb	-	엄지손가락
	tooth	odont(o)-	치아
	tongue	gloss-, glott-	혀
	toe	dactyl(o)-	발가락
	tumour	cel-, onc(o)-	종양
U	ureter	ureter(o)-	요관, 수뇨관
	urethra	urethr(o)-, urethr(a)-	요도
	urine, urinary System	ur(o)-	소변, 배뇨계
	uterine tubes	sarping(o)-	난관
	uterus	hyster(o)-, metr(o)-	자궁
V	vagina	colp(o)-	질
	vein	phleb(o)-	정맥
	vulva	episi(o)-	외음부
	womb	hyster(o)-, metr(o)-	자궁
	wrist	carp(o)-	손목

2. 의료 용어에 쓰이는 접두사/접미사 (list of medical prefixes and suffixes)

	접두사/접미사	의미(영문)	의미(한글)	ex)
A	a-, an-	an absence of, without	-없는	apathy, analgia
	ab-	away from	-로부터 멀리	abduction
	abdomin(o)-	Of or relating to the abdomen	복부와 관련해서	abdomen
	-ac,	pertaining to	-을 포함하는	cardiac
	aesthesio-	sensation	감각	anesthesia
	algia	pain	통증	myalgia
	an-	not, without	없는	analgesia
	an	anus	항문	
	ante-	before, in front of	-앞의, 전방의	antepartum
	anti-	against, opposed to	-에 반해서	antibody
	arteri(o)-	artery	동맥	artery
	arthr(o)-	Joints, limbs	관절, 사지	arthritis
	-ase	enzyme	효소	lactase
	-ation	process	과정	habitation, lubrication
	aur(i)-	ear	귀	aural
	aut(o)	self	자신 스스로	autoimmune
	aux(o)	increase, growth	증가, 증식	auxocardia
B	bi-	twice, double	둘의	binary
	bio-	life	생명	biology
	bronch(i)-	bronchus	기관	bronchiolitis
	bucc(o)-	cheek	뺨	buccolabial
C	capill-	hair	모발	capillus
	capit-	head	머리	capitation
	carcin(o)-	cancer	암	carcinoma
	cardi(o)-	heart	심장	cardiology
	carp(o)-	wrist	손목	carpopedal
	cata-	down, under	-아래	cataract
	cerebr(o)-	brain	뇌	cerebrology
	cervic-	neck, cervix	목, 경부	cervicodosal
	chem(o)-	chemistry	화학	chemotherapy
	chir(o)-	hand	손	chiropractor
	chol(e)-	bile	담즙	cholaemia
	-cidal	killing, destroying	파괴, 박멸	bacteriocidal

	접두사/접미사	의미(영문)	의미(한글)	ex)
C	cili-	eyelash, eyelid	눈썹, 눈꺼풀	ciliary
	circum-	around	둘레	circumcision
	clast	break	파괴	osteoclast
	co-	with, together	-와 함께	coenzymes
	col-	colon	대장	colonoscopy
	colp(o)-	vagina	질	colposcopy
	com-	with, together	-와 함께	coenzyme
	contra	against	-반하는	contraindicate
	coro-	pupil of the eye	눈동자	corectomy
	cordi-	heart	심장	cordis
	coron-	heart	심장	
	cost(o)-	ribs	갈비뼈	costochondral
	cox-	hip, haunch	엉덩이	coxopodite
	crani(o)-	cranium	두개골	craniology
	-crine	to secerete	내분비	endocrine
	cry(o)-	cold	한랭	cryoablation
	cutane-	skin	피부	subcutaneous
	cyt(o)-	cell	세포	cytokine
D	dacryo-	tear	눈물	
	dent-	tooth	치아	dentist
	dermat(o)-	skin	피부	dermatology
	di-	apart, separation	분리	
	dis-	seperation	분리	dissection
	dors(o)-	back	등	dorsal
	-dynia	pain	통증	vulvodynia
	dys-	bad, difficult	나쁜, 어려운	dysphagia
E	-eal	pertaining to	-을 포함하는	
	ect(o)-	outer, outside	밖의	ectopic pregnancy
	-ectasis, -ectasia	expansion, dilation	확대	bronchiectasis
	-ectomy	removal of a body part	절제	mastectomy
	-emesis	vomiting condition	구토 증세	hematemesis
	-emia	blood condition	혈액상태	anemia
	endo-	inside, within	-안에	endocrinology
	enter(o)-	intestine	내장의	gastoenterology
	epi-	on, upon	-위의	epidural
	esthesio-	sensation	감각	
	ex-	out of, away from	-의 밖	exophthalmos

접두사/접미사		의미(영문)	의미(한글)	ex)
E	exo-	outside, external	외부의	exoskeleton
	extra-	outside	외부의	extradural hematoma
F	faci(o)-	face	얼굴	facioplegic
	front-	forehead	이마, 앞이마	frontonasal
G	gastr(o)-	stomach	위	gastric bypass
	-genic	producing	형성하는	cardiogenic shock
	genu-	knee	무릎	genu valgum
	gingiv-	gum	잇몸	gingivitis
	glauc(o)-	bluish-gray color	녹(회)색의	glaucoma
	-gnosis	knowledge	지식	diagnosis
	-gram, -gramme	record or picture	도표	angiogram
	-graph	record data	기록지	electrocardiograph
	-graphy	process of recording	기록함	angiography
	gyno-	woman	여성	gynocology
H	halluc-	to wander in mind	환각	hallucination
	hemat-	blood	혈액	hematology
	hemi-	one-half	반, 2분의 1	cerebral hemisphere
	hepat-	liver	간	hepatology
	hidr(o)	sweat	발한, 땀	hyperhidrosis
	hist(o)	tissue	조직	histology
	hom(o)-	same	동일한	homosexuality
	hydr(o)-	water	수분	hydrophobe
	hyper-	extreme, beyond normal	정상보다 높은	hypertension
	hyp(o)-	below normal	정상보다 낮은	hypotension
	hyster(o)-	womb, uterus	자궁	hysterectomy
I	-i-asis	condition	상태	mydriasis
	-iatry	field in medicine	-학	psychiatry
	-ic	pertaining to	-을 포함하는	hepatic
	inter-	betseen, among	-사이	interarticular
	intra-	within	-안에	intracranial
	-ist	one who specilzes in	전문가	pathologist
	-itis	inflammation	염증	tonsillitis
	isch-	restriction	제한	ischemia
K	kerat(o)-	cornea(eye or skin)	각막	Keratoscope
L	labi(o)-	lip	입술	labiodental
	lacrim(o)-	tear	눈물	lacrimal
	lact(i)-	milk	우유	lactation

접두사/접미사		의미(영문)	의미(한글)	ex)
L	lapar(o)-	abdomen wall	옆구리	laparotomy
	laryng(o)-	larynx	후두	larynx
	latero-	lateral	측면의	lateral pectoral nerve
	-lepsy	attack, seizure	발작	epilepsy
	lip(o)	fat	지방	liposuction
	log(o)-	speech	언어능력	
	-logist	someone who studies certain field	전문가	oncologist
	-logy	study or practice of a certain field	전문학	oncology
	lymph(o)-	lymph	림프	lymphedema
	-lysis	destruction, seperation	마비	paralysis
M	macr(o)-	large, long	큰, 긴	macrophage
	mamm(o)	breast	유방	mammogram
	mammill(o)-	nipple	유두, 젖꼭지	
	manu-	hand	손	manual
	-megaly	enlargement	확대	splenomegaly
	melan(o)-	black color	검정색	melanin
	melos	extremity	사지	erythromelalgia
	mening(o)-	membrane		meningitis
	-metry	process of measuring	측량	optometry
	metr(o)-	uterus	자궁	metrorrhagia
	micro-	small	작은	microscope
	mon(o)-	single	하나뿐인, 한 개의	infectious mononucleosis
	muscul(o)-	muscle	근육	musculoskeletal system
	my(o)-	muscle	근육	myoblast
	myc(o)-	fungus	용종, 균류, 균상종	onychomycosis
	myring(o)-	eardrum	고막	myringotomy
	myx(o)-	mucus	점액	myxoma
N	narc(o)-	numb, sleep	마비, 숙면	narcolepsy
	nas(o)-	nose	코	nasal
	necr(o)-	death	사망	necrotizing fasciitis
	neo-	new	새로운	neoplasm
	nephr(o)-	kidney	신장	Nephrology
	nerv-	nervous system	신경계	nerve
	neur(o)-	nervous system	신경계	Neurifibromatosis
	normo-	normal	정상	normacapnia
O	ocul(o)-	eye	눈	oculist
	odont(o)-	teeth	치아	orthodontist

	접두사/접미사	의미(영문)	의미(한글)	ex)
O	odyn(o)-	pain	통증	stomatodynia
	-oesophageal	gullet	식도	
	om(o)-	shoulder	어깨	omoplate
	onco-	tumor, bulk, volume	종양	Oncology
	oo-	woman's egg	난자	oogenesis
	oophor(o)-	woman's ovay	난소	oophorectomy
	opthalm(o)-	eye	눈	Opthalmology
	optic(o)-	chemical properties of the eye	눈의 화학적 특성	opticochemical
	or(o)-	mouth	입	oral
	orth(o)-	straight, correct	교정	orthpdontist
	-osis	a condition, disease or increase	증세, 병, 진행	osteoporosis
	ost(o)-	bone	뼈, 골	Osteoporosis
	ot(o)-	ear	귀	Otopathy
	ovari(o)-	ovary	난소	
	oxy-	oxygen	산소	
P	para-	abnormal		
	-paresis	slight paralysis	가벼운 마비	hemiparesis
	path(o)-	disease	질병	Pathology
	ped-	foot	발, 족	Pedoscope
	pelv(i)-	hip bone	엉덩이뼈	pelvis
	-penia-	deficiency	결핍	osteopenia
	peo-	penis	음경	Peotomy
	-pepsia	digestion	소화	Dyspepsia
	per-	through	-을 통해	
	peri-	around	둘레	Periodontal
	phagia	relating to eating	섭취	Sacophagia
	phamaco-	drug, medication	약	Phamacology
	-phobia	exaggerated fear, sensitivity	공포	arachnophobia
	phon(o)-	sound	소리	
	phot(o)-	light	빛	Photopathy
	-plasia	fomation, developement	형성, 발달, 성장	Achondroplasia
	-plasty	surgical repair, reconstruction	외과적 수술 교정, 재건	rhinoplasty
	-plegia	paralysis	마비	paraplegia
	pneum(o)-	lungs	폐	Pneumonocyte
	poly-	plurality	복수	Polymyositis
	por(o)-	pore	(피부의) 털구멍	

	접두사/접미사	의미(영문)	의미(한글)	ex)
P	post-	after	-후	postoperation
	pre-	before	-전	prematurity
	prim-	most important	가장 중요한	primary
	pro-	before	-전	procephalic
	psych(o)-	mind	마음	Psycology
	psor-	itching	가려움	Psoriasis
	pulmon-	lung	폐	Pulmonary
	pyel(o)-	pevis	골반	Pyelonephritis
	pyo-	pus	고름	Pyometra
	pyro-	fever	열	Antipyretic
Q	quadr(i)-	four	넷, 4	quadriceps
R	radio-	radiation	방사선	radiowave
	re-	again	재, 다시	relapse
	rect(o)-	rectum	직장	
	ren(o)-	kidney	신장	renal
	retro	backward	역류	retroversion
	rhachi(o)-	spine	척추	rachial
	rhin(o)-	nose	코	rhinoplasty
	-rrhagia	rapid flow of blood	빠른 혈액 흐름	
	-rrhpha	surgical suturing	수술적 봉합	
	-rrhea	flowing, discharge	흐름, 배출	Diarrhea
	-rrhexis	rupture	파열	
	-rrhoea	flowing, discharge	흐름, 배출	diarrhoea
S	schiz(o)-	split, double -sided	분열	schzophrenia
	scler(o)-	hardness	경직	atherosclerosis
	-sclerosis	hardening of the skin	피부의 경직	Multiple sclerosis
	scoli(o)-	twisted	뒤틀린	scoliosis
	-scope	instrument for viewing	-경(기구)	endoscope
	scopy	use of instrument of viewing	내시경(시술)	endoscopy
	semi-	one-half, partly	반	
	sigmoid(o)-	sigmoid colon	s상 결장	
	sinus-	sinus	누, 공동	Sinusitis
	somat(o)-	body	신체	
	spasmo-	spasm	경련	Spasmodic dysphonia
	splen(o)-	spleen	비장	splenectomy
	spondyl(o)-	vertebra	척추	Spondylitis
	-stasis	stop, stand	멈춤	

	접두사/접미사	의미(영문)	의미(한글)	ex)
S	steth(o)-	pertaining to the upper chest, chest, the area above the breast and under the neck	흉부	Stethoscope
	stom(a)	mouth	입	stomatitis
	sub-	beneth	아래	subcutaneous tissue
	supra-	above, excessive	위의, 과도한	supraorbital
T	-tension	pressure	압력	Hypertension
	therm(o)-	heat	온열	
	thorac(i)-	pertaining to the upper chest, chest, the area above the breast and under the neck	흉부	thorax
	thromb(o)-	blood clot	혈전	thrombus
	thyr(o)-	thyroid	갑상선	thyroiditis
	thym(o)-	emotions	감정	dysthimia
	-tomy	incision	절개	Gastrotomy
	-tony	tension	긴장	
	tox(i)-	toxin	독	detoxification
	trache(o)-	trachea	기관	
	trichi(o)-	hair	모발	tricocyst
	-trophy	nourishment	영양상태, 양육	
	tympan(o)-	eardrum	고막	Tympanocentesis
U	umblic-	umbilicus	탯줄	umblical
	ungui-	nail	손톱	ungiform
	un(i)-	one		unilateral
	ur(o)-	urine	소변	Urology
	urico-	uric acid	요산	
	urin-	urinary system	배뇨 기관	uriniferous
	uter(o)-	womb	자궁	uterus
V	vagin-	vagina	질	vagina
	varic(o)-	vein	혈관	varicose
	ven-	vein	혈관	vein
	ventr(o)-	belly	배꼽	ventrodosal
	ventricul(o)-	ventricles	심실	cardiac ventriculography
	-version	turning	전환	anteversion
X	xer(o)-	dry, desert-like	마른, 건조한	Xerostomia
Y	-y	condition or process of	과정	sugery
Z	zym(o)-	enzyme	효소	

3. 색(color)에 대한 용어

표현	어원	의미
black	melano-	검정색
blue	cyano-	파랑색
gray, grey	polio-	회색
green	chlor(o)-	녹색
purple	porphyr(o)-	보라색
red	erythr(o)-, rhod(o)-	적색
red-yellow	cirrh(o)-	적갈색
white	leuc-, leuk-	백색
yellow	xanth(o)-	황색

4. 표현(description)에 대한 크기, 모양, 강도 등 (size, shape, strength, etc.)

표현	어원	의미
bad, incorrect	cac(o)-, dys-	틀린
bent, crooked	ankyl(o)-	굽은
big	mega-, megal(o)-	큰
biggest	megist-	가장 큰
broad, wide	eury-	넓은
cold	cry(o)-	찬
dead	necr(o)-	사망한
equal	is(o)-	동일한
false	pseud(o)-	잘못된
female, feminine	thely-	여성
flat	platy-	납작한
good, well	eu-	좋은
great	mega-, megal(o)-	큰
hard	scler(o)-	딱딱한
heavy	bar(o)-	무거운
hollow	coel(o)-	속이 빈
huge	megal(o)-	커다란
incorrect, bad	cac(o)-, dys-	틀린, 오류의
irregular	poikil(o)	일정치 않은
large, extremely large	mega-	큰, 대형의
largest	megist-	가장 큰
long	macr(o)-	긴
male, masculine	arseno-	남성의
narrow	sten(o)-	좁은
new	neo-	새로운
normal, correct	orth(o)-	정상의
old	paleo-	오랜
sharp	oxy-	날카로운
short	brachy-	짧은
small	micr(o)-	작은
smallest	-	가장 작은
slow	brady-	느린
fast	tachy-	빠른

표현	어원	의미
soft	malac(o)-	무른
straight	orth(o)-	곧은, 똑바른
thick	pachy-	두꺼운
varied, various	poikilo-	다양한
well, good	eu-	좋은
wide, broad	eury-	넓은

5. 위치(position)에 대한 표현

표현	어원	의미
around	peri-	둘레
left	levo-	왼쪽
middle	mes(o)-	중간
right	dexi(o)-	오른쪽
surrounding	peri-	주위

6. 양(amount, quantity)에 대한 표현

표현	어원	의미
double	diplo-	이중의, 두 배의
equal	iso-	동등한
few	oligo-	적은
half	hemi-	반
many, much	poly-	많은
twice	dis-	두 배의

7. 미국 의료보험과 관계있는 용어

미국인으로 우리나라 의료기관을 찾는 환자들에는 실제 치료와 관광을 목적으로 하는 미국인과 현재 국내에 거주하고 있는 미국인, 그리고 미국에 거주하는 해외 동포들이 있다. 이들은 대부분 미국에서 가입한 보험을 갖고 있는데 현재 국내 몇몇 병원에서는 이러한 보험사와 계약을 체결하는 등 외국인 유치에 노력을 기하고 있다.

이에 따라, 의료기관에서는 보험 회사와의 협약을 통해, 보험 가입자인 환자의 치료비 등을 청구하는 과정이 필요 불가결하게 되었다.

여기에서는 건강보험에 관련된 기본적인 단어들을 정리해서 그 의미들을 이해하여, 보험사 관계의 사무적 처리에 활용하도록 하였다.

Agent	중개인, 대리점
In the insurance industry, an agent is appointed by an insurance company to sell insurance policies. The agent represents the insurance company, not the insured.	건강보험 회사를 대행해 주는 중개인으로 건강보험을 고객들에게 판매하는 일을 한다.
Assignment	지정, 위탁
Your signed authorization to your doctor or hospital (medical provider) assigning payment to be made directly to them for your medical treatment.	환자가 동의서에 서명함으로써 치료비가 의료기관 및 의료진에게 직접 지불되도록 지정해 주는 것을 의미한다.
Banding	무리, 일단
Organizing people together by age groups to calculate premiums.	의료 보험비 책정 고객을 연령별로 그룹으로 나누는 일을 말한다.
Broker	중개인, 알선자
A person licensed by the State to sell insurance coverage with multiple health plans or insurers. The broker represents you and not the insurance companies. The broker helps you shop for the best policy.	여러 가지 다양한 건강보험사 또는 건강보험에 대한 정보를 갖고 고객들의 입장에 서서 각자에게 가장 적합한 보험을 권해 주고 가입할 수 있도록 도와주는 중개인이다. 이들은 보험 회사를 대표하는 입장이 아니고 고객들의 입장에서 보험 가입을 도와준다.
Business Day	영업일
Every day that insurance companies are open for business, which excludes Saturday, Sunday, and state and federal holidays.	보험사가 업무를 하는 날들을 일컬어 비즈니스 데이라고 한다. 미국의 경우 토요일, 일요일, 그리고 연방 정부, 주 정부에서 지정하는 공휴일은 업무를 보지 않는다.

Capitation	**인원별 할당**
A flat per patient fee paid to providers no matter how many services they have provided	치료를 받은 횟수와 관계없이 환자 한 명당 제공자에게 균일하게 지불해야 하는 금액
Certificate of Coverage	**보상 범위에 대한 증명**
A document issued to a member of a group health insurance plan showing evidence of participation in the insurance	보험 가입자에게 발급되는 보험의 보상 내용에 대한 증명서
Certificate of Creditable Coverage	**신용 보상 범위**
A written statement from your prior insurance company or health plan documenting the length of time you were covered	이전에 가입해 있던 건강보험사가 작성한 고객의 보험 가입 기간에 대한 내용 기록서
Chronic Condition	**만성병, 만성 증세**
A medical condition or disease that goes on for a long period of time. Examples are diabetes and cystic fibrosis.	장기간에 걸친 만성적인 증상이나 질환. 예를 들어 당뇨병, 낭포성 섬유증이 있다.
Claim	**요구, 청구**
A notification to your insurance company that payment is due under the policy provisions.	보험 회사에 보험 정책에 준해서 치료비를 청구한다는 의미이다.
Coinsurance	**공동보험**
Once you have met your deductible, you pay coinsurance for additional medical care. It is a percentage of the billed charge. For example, your insurance company might pay 80%, and then you would pay 20%. It is similar to a co-pay, but is a percentage instead of a dollar amount.	환자가 공제금액(deductible)을 다 지불하고나면 추가적 진료에 대해 공동 보험금을 지불하여야 하는데, 이는 치료비의 일부를 환자가 지불하는 것이다. 예를 들어 치료비의 80%는 보험사가, 20%는 환자가 지불하는 보험 정책이다.
Co-payment	**사용자 부담지불**
The portion of charges you pay to your provider for covered health care services in addition to any deductible. For example, $20 for an office visit or $15 for a prescription drug. It is similar to coinsurance, but it is a dollar amount instead of a percentage of the charges.	공제금액 외에 환자가 의료기관에 진료를 받을 때마다 일정 금액을 지불하는 것을 말한다. 예를 들어 의사 방문 때마다 20달러씩, 처방약을 살 때마다 15달러씩 지불하는 등의 정책이다. coinsurance는 어떤 비율을 지불하는 것이고, copayment는 일정금액을 지불하는 것이다.
Coverage	**보상**
The scope of protection provided by an insurance contract which includes any of the listed benefits in an insurance policy	보험 정책에 등록되어 있는 보험계약에 의해 공급된 보호영역
Creditable Coverage or Prior Qualifying Coverage	**신용 보상 범위**

The number of months you had health insurance in place before your current or new policy became effective. Creditable coverage must be counted towards any pre-existing condition exclusion in either an individual or group policy.	현재 혹은 새로 가입한 보험이 유효하게 되기까지의 기간을 말한다. 이는 개인 가입자에게나 단체 가입자에게나 가입 이전에 있던 증세에 대해 보험금 지급을 제외시키고자 하는 데 목적이 있다.
Deductible	**공제금액**
The amount you must pay for medical services each year before your insurance begins paying.	환자가 매년 정해진(가입한 보험 정책에 따라 다른) 금액을 치료비로 지불하는 것을 일컫는 말이다. 매년 정해진 금액이 될 때까지 환자는 의료비를 자신이 지불하고 그 금액이 넘어가면서 보험사의 지불이 시작된다.
Denial	**거절**
An insurance company decision to withhold a claim payment or preauthorization. A denial may be made because the medical service is not covered, not medically necessary, or experimental or investigational.	치료비 청구나 사전위임에 대해 보험사가 거절하는 것을 의미한다. 보험 보상범위에 속하지 않는 진료이거나 의학적으로 필요 없는 진료이거나 또는 실험적 혹은 연구를 위한 진료일 경우에 의료비 지불을 거절하게 된다.
Drug Formulary	**약 처방서**
A list of drugs that an insurer will pay for. Drugs that are not on the formulary ("off-formulary") are sometimes covered but are more expensive (see "excluded drugs"). To you, the cheapest drugs are generic drugs that are on the formulary, and the most expensive drugs are name-brand drugs that are off-formulary.	보험사가 지불해 주는 약의 종류들 목록이다. 이 목록에 제외된 약도 때로 보험사가 지불해 주기도 하지만 좀 더 비싸다. 환자에게 가장 저렴하게 약을 구입하는 방법은, 목록에 있는 일반 명칭으로 판매되는 약(generic drug)을 구입하는 것이고, 목록에 없는, 상표 있는 약(name-brand drug)을 구입하는 경우가 가장 비싸게 구입하게 되는 경우이다.
Elimination Period	**제외 기간**
A period of time before benefits are payable	보험비가 지급될 수 있을 때 이전의 기간
Evidence-Based Medicine	**증명된 약**
In evidence-based medicine, treatment success is measured by a careful study of the outcome, using both the clinical expertise of the provider, as well as the most up-to-date research available.	증명된 약, 치료의 성공은 결과를 전문치료사의 기술과 최신의 연구결과를 바탕으로 하는 고찰을 통해 조심스럽게 결정된다.
Excluded Drugs	**제외되는 약들**
Drugs not covered by the insurance policy	보험에서 지불해 주지 않는 약들
Exclusions and/or Limitations	**제외 그리고/혹은 제한**
Conditions or circumstances spelled out in an insurance policy which limit or exclude coverage benefits. It is important to read all exclusion,	보험사 보상에서 제외되거나 제한되는 증상들이나 상황들. 보험사의 정책에 관해서, 그리고 보상 범위에 대한 규정에 대해서 자세

limitation, and reduction clauses in your health insurance policy or certificate of coverage to determine which expenses are not covered.	히 검토하여 제외, 제한 그리고 감면 등에 대한 내용을 파악하고 있어야 한다.
Experimental and/or Investigational Medical Services	**실험적 그리고/혹은 연구를 위한 의료서비스**
A drug, device, procedure, treatment plan, or other therapy which is currently not within the accepted standards of medical care	현재 의료적 치료의 범위에 벗어나는 약, 기구, 처치, 치료 계획 혹은 다른 치료요법
Fee-for-Service	**서비스 요금**
A system in which you pay the provider for each single service or procedure	각각의 치료나 처치에 대해 의료진에게 지불하는 제도
Generic Drug	**상표 없는 약품(상표등록이 되어 있지 않은 약)**
A drug that is similar to a name-brand drug but not covered by original patents and therefore cheaper. For example, the generic for the name-brand "Vicodin®" is "hydrocodone." If you buy a generic drug, you usually pay less co-pay.	상표가 등록되어 있지는 않지만 상표가 등록된 약과 유사하고 그래서 값이 저렴한 약. 예를 들어 바이코딘이라는 상품명을 가진 약은 하이드로코돈이라는 유사약이 있다. 이런 유사약을 구입할 경우 공동보험료를 적게 낸다.
Grace Period	**유예 기간**
A specified period immediately following the premium due date during which a payment can be made to continue a policy in force without interruption. This applies only to Life and Health policies. Check your policy to be sure that a grace period is offered and how many days, if any, are allowed.	보험료 지불 기간이 지난 이후 특정 기간을 지불 유예 기간으로 정해서 보험의 유효함을 지속시켜 주는 것이다. 이것은 단지 생명 보험과 건강보험에만 적용이 된다. 환자는 보험사가 지불 유예 기간을 주는지, 그리고 며칠간을 주는지 등에 대해 알아보아야 한다.
Group Health Plan	**단체 건강보험**
When groups of individuals are covered under one insurance contract. Usually people are offered group health plans by their employers.	어떤 단체의 개개인이 한 보험에 가입해 있는 경우이다. 보통 고용주에 의해 (직장 등) 보험에 가입하는 경우이다.
Home Health Care	**가정 건강 관리**
Health care provided in your home	환자의 주거지에서 제공되는 건강관리
Hospice Care	**호스피스 관리**
Care given to someone expected to live less than six months due to a terminal disease or condition. Hospice care can be given at home or in a hospice center or a board and care facility.	말기적 질병이나 증세로 6개월 이내에 사망할 환자 진료를 말한다. 호스피스 관리는 집이나 호스피스 시설, 기숙과 진료를 병행하는 시설 등에서 이루어진다.
Independent Medical Review (IMR)	**독립된 의료적 검토**
A process where expert medical professionals, who have no relationship to your health insurance company or health plan, review specific medical	보험 회사나 보험 제도 등과 관계가 없는 의학 전문가들이 보험사의 결정들에 대해 검토하는 것을 말한다.

decisions made by the insurance company. California law provides for an Independent Medical Review (IMR) program depending upon what type of coverage you have.

미국 캘리포니아 주에서는 어떤 보상 범위인지에 따라 이 제도를 법으로 허용하고 있다.

Individual Health Plan | **개인 보험 정책**

A form of health insurance designed to cover just one person (and often immediate family members), as opposed to someone covered by a group plan

한 개인을 위해 고안된 건강보험
단체 건강 보험과 상응하는 보험

Insurance Company | **보험 회사**

An insurance company must be licensed by the Department of Insurance to sell health insurance. The insurer issues policies which outline coverage. An insurance policy is a contract between the insured and the insurance company. You pay your premiums to an insurance company. They then pay some or all of your medical provider's bills when you need treatment.

보험 회사는 관계 기관에 등록이 되어 있어야 하며, 보험의 보상 범위를 정한다. 보험 정책은 보험사와 가입자간의 계약 체결이다. 가입자는 의료 보험비를 보험사에 지불한다. 그리고 보험사는 가입자의 진료비의 전부 혹은 일부를 지불해 준다.

Insured | **가입자**

The person, group, or organization whose life, health or property is covered by an insurance policy

생명, 건강, 소유물 등에 대한 보험에 가입한 개인, 단체 혹은 기관

Lifetime Limit | **보험한계지불**

A dollar limit on how much the insurance company will pay in your lifetime. An insurer may, for example, cover up to $1 million over your lifetime. Above this they will pay nothing.

보험사가 개인의 일생을 통해 지불하는 금액의 범위. 예를 들어 보험사가 개인 당 100만 달러가 그 한계 지불액이다. 그 이상 초과되는 금액은 지불하지 않는다.

Long-term Care | **장기 진료**

Long Term Care is the assistance or supervision you may need when you are not able to do some of the basic "activities of daily living" (ADL) like bathing, dressing or moving from a bed to a chair. Examples of conditions in which you might need assistance with ADLs are: injury, illness, advanced age, or mental deterioration.

환자가 목욕, 옷입기, 침대에서 일어나 의자로 가는 등의 일상생활을 하기 어려울 때 도움이나 관리를 받고 생활하게 되는 것을 말한다. 중상, 병, 노화, 또는 정신적 퇴화 등이 일상적 활동을 불가능하게 만드는 원인들이다.

Managed Care | **경영 관리**

Managed care generally emphasizes cost control and may provide coverage for preventive medicine. There are restrictions on the types of procedures that can be used for each medical condition. The amounts that can be charged for

의료비용을 줄이기 위한 경영을 하고, 또 그의 일환으로 예방약을 공급한다. 각각의 증상에 따라 시행되는 진료에 대해 지불되는 비용을 제한한다. 진료에 따라 정해진 금액은 보험의 기간, 조건에 따라 결정된다.

the procedures are described by the terms and conditions of the plan.	
Major Medical Plan	**주요 의료 보험**
A high-limit, high deductible plan to cover catastrophic illness or injury. Major medical used to be called "catastrophic insurance."	극심한 병 혹은 상해 등을 보상해 주는 보상비 제한과 연 공제 금액이 높이 책정되어 있는 보험. '재해 보험'이라고 불렸었다.
Medically Necessary	**의학적인 필요성**
A drug, device, procedure, treatment plan, or other therapy that is covered under your health insurance policy and that your doctor, hospital, or provider has determined essential for your medical well-being, specific illness, or underlying condition	보험에서 보상해 주거나 혹은 의사, 병원, 또는 그 외 의료서비스 제공자가 환자의 건강, 특정 병 혹은 잠재적 증상에 대해 필요하다고 결정하는 모든 약, 기구, 처치, 치료 계획 혹은 다른 치료 요법
Name-brand Drug	**고유 상품명 의약품**
A drug sold under a name-brand, and covered by original patents. Name-brand drugs are more expensive than generic drugs, and you usually have a higher co-pay for them than generics.	특허법에 등록되어 있고 고유 상품명을 가진 약품들. 이런 약들은 등록 상표가 없는 유사 약들에 비해 값이 비싸고, 공동 지불액이 더 많다.
Open Enrollment	**개방 등록**
The time (usually a preset two-week or one-month period annually) when you can change health plans under your employer's group plan	고용주의 단체 보험 아래서 개인의 보험 정책을 변경할 수 있는 기간(보통 2주일 기간이 책정되고, 일 년에 한 달 정도의 기간이다)
Over-the-Counter Drug	**일반의약품(OTC 약품)**
You don't need a prescription to obtain over-the-counter drugs	의사의 처방 필요 없이 구입할 수 있는 약들
Out-of-Pocket	**환자비용**
The amount of money you pay for medical services after insurance has paid its contribution.	보험사에서 지불한 후 환자가 지불해야 하는 나머지 금액
Out-of-Pocket Maximum	**최대 환자 비용**
The most you will have to pay in a year for deductibles and coinsurance for covered benefits	환자가 일 년간 지불하는 공제금액과 공동 지불금의 최대치
Plan (Group) Number	**보험그룹 번호**
Insurance has different program which is designed for the customer's need.	개인마다 다른 조건에 맞는 여러 가지 형태의 보험이 있다.
Policy	**보험 정책**
The written contract between an individual or group policyholder and an insurance company. The policy outlines the duties, obligations, and responsibilities of both the policyholder and the	개인 혹은 단체 보험 가입자와 보험사 간의 계약 조건을 기록한 것이다. 보험 가입자와 보험사의 의무, 협정, 책임 등을 내용으로 한다. 계약 조건의 내용, 그에 따라 제한되는

insurance company. A policy may include any application, endorsement, certificate, or any other document that can describe, limit, or exclude coverage benefits under the policy.	사항, 제외되는 사항 등의 적용, 승인, 증명 혹은 그 외 모든 서류 등도 포함한다.
Portability	**보험금통산제**
The ability to purchase individual health insurance without being denied of coverage because of a pre-existing condition	이전에 갖고 있는 증상으로 인해 제한 없이 개인이 보험에 가입할 수 있는 자격
Pre-authorization	**사전 승인**
Some insurance companies require authorization from them before they will pay for medical services like hospitalization or surgery.	몇몇 보험 회사는 입원이나 수술에 앞서 보험 회사의 사전 승인을 받도록 규정하고 있다.
Pre-existing Condition	**사전에 있었던 증세**
Any illness or health condition for which you have received medical advice or treatment during the six months prior to obtaining health insurance. Group healthcare policies cover pre-existing conditions after you have been insured for six months, and individual policies cover pre-existing conditions after you have been insured for one year. Creditable coverage must be counted towards any pre-existing condition exclusion in either an individual or group policy.	보험에 가입하기 전 6개월 이내에 의료적 진단이나 치료를 받았던 어떤 질병이나 증세. 단체 가입자의 경우 가입 후 6개월이 지나면 그리고 개인 가입자의 경우 가입 후 1년이 지나면 사전에 있던 증세들에 대해서도 보상받을 수 있게 된다. 개인이나 단체 가입자에게나 사전에 있었던 증세 중 제외되는 규제 내용에 영향을 받게 된다.
Premium	**보험비**
The money you pay for health insurance	가입자 개인이 부담해야 하는 비용
Prescription Drug	**처방약**
You must have a doctor's prescription to receive a prescription drug.	처방약은 의사의 처방전이 있어야만 구입할 수 있다.
Preventive Medicine	**예방약**
Health care designed to prevent disease or discover and treat disease in the early stage. Examples: Annual physical exam, PAP Smear, cholesterol screening, mammography, infant vaccination, etc.	의료진은 질병을 예방하거나 조기 발견과 치료에 중점을 두고자 노력한다. 예를 들어 연중 신체검사, 자궁암 검사, 콜레스테롤 수치 검사, 유방암 검사, 어린이 예방접종 등이 이런 예방 의료서비스에 속한다.
Primary Care Physician	**주치의**
Your Primary Care Physician ("PCP") is the doctor you choose to provide basic health care. In an HMO, your PCP must refer you to a specialist if you need to see one.	기본 건강 치료를 위해 찾는 의사를 일컫는다. 미국 보험제도의 HMO 혹은 PCP 제도는 전문가에게 가려면 주치의의 추천(referral)이 필요하다.

Provider | **의료서비스 제공자**

Any person or place that provides health care or prescription drugs. Providers can be doctors, hospitals, pharmacies, chiropractors, etc.

치료나 처방약을 제공하는 개인 혹은 의료기관. 의사, 병원, 약국, 척추 교정 지압 요법 전문가 등이다.

Rating Facrtors | **등급 요인들**

Health insurance premiums are calculated using many rating factors. Rating factors have much more influence on individual policy premiums than on group polices. Rating factors can include:

- Age: the older you are, the more you might pay.
- Health: the poorer your health, the more you might pay.
- Chronic conditions: having one or more chronic or existing conditions can increase your premium.
- Smoking/alcohol use: some companies charge more if you use tobacco or alcohol.
- Gender: some insurance plans charge more depending upon your gender.
- Geographic region: companies break-down coverage areas into 6-8 regions. Which region you live in can affect your premium.

보험 가입자의 등급을 정하는 데 영향을 끼치는 요인들이다. 이런 요인들은 단체보다는 개인 가입자에게 더 많은 영향을 끼친다.

- 나이(age): 나이가 많을수록 수가가 올라간다.
- 건강(health): 건강 상태가 나쁠수록 수가가 올라간다.
- 만성질환(chronic conditions): 한 가지 혹은 그 이상의 만성질환 환자인 경우 수가가 올라간다.
- 흡연/알코올(smoking/alcohol use): 흡연자이거나 알코올 소비자의 경우 수가 올라간다.
- 성별(gender): 회사에 따라 성별에 따라 달리 책정된다.
- 지리학적 위치(geographic region): 가입자가 어디에 거주하는지에 따라 다르게 책정한다.

Small Employer | **작은 기업주**

In California's insurance code, a small employer is anyone who employs from 2-50 people. The employer(s) can be included in this number.

미국 캘리포니아 주에서는 작은 기업이란 2~50명의 고용자가 있는 기업을 일컫는다. 이 숫자에 고용주도 포함한다.

Social Security Number | **사회보장번호**

Social Security number is given to US citizen and residents to get a job, and collect Social Security benefits and receive some other government services. SSS number is 9 digit number.

미국 시민권자, 영주권자에게 주는 사회보장번호이며, 직장을 갖거나 사회보장 혜택을 받는 등 정부가 제공하는 서비스를 받을 수 있는 권한을 갖게 해준다. 9개의 숫자로 이루어져 있다.

Stop-Loss | **손실 중지**

An insurer may pay 100% of covered benefit charges after you have met your deductible and coinsurance requirements, and your out-of-pocket maximum.

가입자가 공제액, 공동 지불액, 그리고 지불 최대 금액을 지불하고 난 후의 모든 금액은 보험사가 지불한다.

Third-Party Payer	제3지불자
Anyone who pays for health care other than you. Usually your insurance company. When an insurer contracts with an entity to pay on their behalf.	환자 자신이 아닌 제3자가 진료비를 지불하는 경우이다. 보통 보험사를 말한다. 보험사가 지불에 대한 계약을 이행하는 것이다.
Utilization Review	**이용조사**
Insurance companies and hospitals watch their costs and quality by having medical personnel review selected medical cases. They look at the types and frequency of medical services given and the charges associated with them.	보험사와 병원은 여러 가지 치료 내용을 의료 전문가를 통해, 검토하게 함으로써 비용과 질에 대해 통제한다. 그들은 치료 방안, 치료 빈도, 치료비 책정 등을 검토한다.

참고문헌

이우주, 1990, 『의학대사전』, 아카데미서적.

Lea M. Sims, 2002, *The Book of Style for Medical Transcription*, Association for Healthcare Documentation Integrity.

Marcy O. Diehl, 1979, *Medical Transcription Techniques and Procedures*, SAUNDERS.

http://www.medicalmutual.com/risk/forms/pocedure_consent.pdf:consent to medical/Surgical Procedure

http://racing.ussailing.org/Assets/Racing/JO/safety_medical_consent_form.pdf:Medical Consent Form

http://www.ossur.com/lisalib/getfile.aspx?itemid

http://sites.google.com/site/medicaltranscriptionsamples/soap-note-chart-note-progress-note-medical-transcription-transcribed-sample

http://www.haustranscription.com/gyn.htm

http://policies.ncsu.edu/regulation/reg-11-45-6

http://en.wikipedia.org/wiki/List_of_medical_roots,_suffixes_and_prefixes

http://www.insurance.ca.gov/0100-consumers/0070-health-issues/health-insurance-terms.cfm

http://en.wikipedia.org/wiki/Medical_record

http://www.nlm.nih.gov/medlineplus

http://www.enotes.com/nursing-encyclopedia/medical-chart

http://www.medical-transcription-online-training.com/tutor3.html

http://www.themtassist.com/medical-transcription-course/medical-transcription-terms/

http://www.mtworld.com/career/BecomeaMedTrans.html

http://www.haustranscription.com/medical_chart.htm

지은이 소개

주영탁

1977~1981 이화여자대학교 생활미술학과를 졸업하고

1981~1982 Rhode Island School of Design에서 MAE(Master in Art Education)를 취득했다.

1985년 미국으로 이민하여,

1989년 St. Francis Medical Center Internal Medicine Clinic에서 매니저로 일하며 의료통역의 일들도 담당했다.

2003년부터 전문 의료 통역사로 여러 의료기관에서 일하기 시작하였으며,

2009년 9월부터 현재까지 한림대 의료관광인재양성센터에서 영어권 의료 용어, 의료관광 서류의 작성과 번역을 강의하고 있다.

저서로 『영어권 의료 용어』(2011, 소화)가 있다.

영어권 의료관광 서류의 번역과 작성

초판 발행 2012년 1월 27일

지은이 주영탁
펴낸이 고화숙
펴낸곳 도서출판 소화
등록 제13-412호
주소 서울시 영등포구 영등포동 7가 94-97
전화 02-2677-5890
팩스 02-2636-6393
홈페이지 www.sowha.com

ISBN 978-89-8410-424-2 93740

값 17,000원

잘못된 책은 언제나 바꾸어 드립니다.